P. Hohenberger · K. Conlon (Eds.)

Staging Laparoscopy

W0050569

Springer
Berlin
Heidelberg
New York
Barcelona
Hong Kong
London
Milan
Paris
Tokyo

P. HOHENBERGER · K. CONLON (Eds.)

Staging Laparoscopy

With 47 Figures, 18 in Color

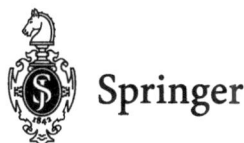 Springer

Prof. Dr. PETER HOHENBERGER
Humboldt University
Division of Surgery and Surgical Oncology
Charité, Robert-Roessle Hospital
Lindenberger Weg 80
13222 Berlin, Germany

KEVIN CONLON, MD, MBA, FACS
Gastric & Mixed Tumor Service
Memorial Sloan-Kettering Cancer Center
1275 York Avenue
New York, NY 10021, USA

ISBN 978-3-642-63000-2   ISBN 978-3-642-56290-7 (eBook)
DOI 10.1007/978-3-642-56290-7

Libary of Congress Cataloging in-Publication Data applied for

Die Deutsche Bibliothek – CIP-Einheitsaufnahme

Staging laparoscopy / Hohenberger, Peter; Conlon, Kevin. – Berlin; Heidelberg;
New York; Barcelona; Hongkong; London; Milan; Paris; Singapore; Tokyo:
Springer, 2002

http://www.springer.de

© Springer-Verlag Berlin Heidelberg 2002
Originally published by Springer-Verlag Berlin Heidelberg New York in 2002
Softcover reprint of the hardcover 1st edition 2002

Production: PRO EDIT GmbH, 69126 Heidelberg, Germany
Cover Design: E. Kirchner, Heidelberg
Typesetting / Reproduction: AM-productions GmbH,
69168 Wiesloch, Germany

Printed on acid-free paper
SPIN: 10690970   24/3130So-5 4 3 2 1 0 -

For Ralph

To Jennifer, Lucy, Caroline and Elizabeth,
whose support never wavers.

Preface

The modern achievement of minimally invasive surgery has focussed primarily on the treatment of benign disease. Consequently, cholecystectomy, hernia repair, and fundoplication represent the overwhelming majority of laparoscopic procedures. Historically, however, the "keyhole" access to the abdominal cavity was intended to assess tumor spread or liver pathology. Creating a pneumoperitoneum has enabled surgeons to explore thoroughly specific areas of the abdomen such as the lesser sac, the subdiaphragmatic liver surface, or the lymph nodes at the celiac axis. As a logical consequence, operative laparoscopy for purposes of staging malignancies related to the abdominal cavity has gained more and more attention.

This book, which represents a joint effort, intends to summarize the rationale, operative technique, and algorithm of laparoscopic staging for cancer:
- It merges different approaches by various medical specialities such as surgical oncologists, gynecologists, urologists, and even medical oncologists.
- It combines the international experience of centers dedicated to the concept of staging laparoscopy. The result is a transatlantic effort fueled from the USA (Memorial Sloan-Kettering Cancer Center, New York) and from central Europe (Berlin, Munich, Frankfurt)

In this book, we focus mainly on technical aspects, indications, and algorithms of staging laparoscopy. Operative techniques do not become outdated very rapidly. Treatment results, however, are published more in current peer-reviewed journals, and it was not our aim to reproduce these results. Thus, we provide a dual view and have specifically not tried to avoid dual-view information. Indications for staging laparoscopy and using laparoscopic ultrasound may be viewed differently in various scientific communities. The chapters of this volume (for example, those on gastric cancer and urological tumors) are independent and may be directed to a different readership in Europe and the USA. Clearly, different techniques are presented and diverse scenarios of intra- and perioperative management are displayed.

We sincerely feel that staging laparoscopy represents a major advantage in the modern management of patients with cancer. Pretreatment staging can be based on histological findings, even regarding nodal status, and must not rely solely on imaging findings. Staging laparoscopy offers a "one-stop shopping" strategy when compared to multistep imaging of a suspected cancer and assessment of its spread. Particularly when considering a neoadjuvant treatment option (in patients with cancer of the esophagus, stomach, or rectum), it is of crucial importance to differentiate between patients with a locally advanced tumor who are candidates for combined modality therapy and those with metastatic tumor spread with treatment aiming for palliation. Staging laparoscopy is not an operation for beginners because it requires an experienced surgical oncologist to assess the decisive steps of judging resectablity and tumor spread.

We conclude from the contributions to this book that during the management of patients with cancer of the abdominal cavity or retroperitoneal space, it is important to aim at a carefully performed staging laparoscopy with laparoscopic ultrasound applications using the methods and techniques as described.

We are grateful to the Deutsche Forschungsgemeinschaft for supporting an International Workshop hosting the protagonists of laparoscopic staging. We also feel indebted to Stephanie Benko and Constanze Sonntag from Springer-Verlag, who continuously supported the idea of this book and made it happen.

Berlin, New York, May 2002   PETER HOHENBERGER,
                                  KEVIN CONLON

Contents

Basic Aspects

Extended Diagnostic Laparoscopy in Gastric Cancer
H. FEUSSNER, S.J.M. KRAEMER, J.R. SIEWERT

Laparoscopic Staging for Pancreatic Malignancy
N.J. ESPAT, K.C. CONLON

Laparoscopic Ultrasonography for Staging of Gastrointestinal Cancer
M. HÜNERBEIN, B. RAU, P. HOHENBERGER

Further Results and Strategies of Clinical Application

Contribution to Initial Staging and Assessment of Treatment Results in Gynecologic Cancers
J.P. CURTIN

Indications in Urologic Tumors
P. RUSSO

Is There Any Role for the Laparoscopic Staging of Urologic Malignancies?
P. FORNARA, C. DOEHN, D. JOCHAM

Impact of Laparoscopy in Malignant Lymphomas
G.B. MANN, K.C. CONLON

Contributors

BANK, W.
Department of General and Vascular Surgery
Johann Wolfgang Goethe University
Theodor-Stern Kai 7, 60590 Frankfurt/Main, Germany

CONLON, K.C.
Director, Endosurgical Program, Department of Surgery,
Memorial Sloan-Kettering Cancer Center, 1275 York Avenue,
New York, NY 10021, USA

CURTIN, J.P.
Gynecology Service, Department of Surgery, Memorial Sloan-
Kettering Cancer Center, 1275 York Avenue, New York, New York
10021, USA

DOEHN, C.
Department of Urology, Medical University of Lübeck, Ratzeburger Allee 160, 23538 Lübeck, Germany

FEUSSNER, H.
Department of Surgery , Klinikum rechts der Isar, Technische
Universität München, Ismaningerstr. 22, 81675 Munich, Germany

FORNARA, P.
Prof. and Chairman of the Urological Department and Trans-
plantation Unit of the Martin-Luther-University Halle-Witten-
berg, Magdeburger Straße 16, 06112 Halle, Germany

GUTT, C.N.
Department of General and Vascular Surgery
Johann Wolfgang Goethe University
60590 Frankfurt/Main, Theodor-Stern Kai 7, Germany

HOHENBERGER, P.

University Hospital Charité, Campus Berlin Buch,
Robert-Roessle Hospital and Tumor Institute,
Humboldt University at Berlin,
Lindenberger Weg 80, 13122 Berlin, Germany

HÜNERBEIN, M.

Division of Surgery and Surgical Oncology, Charitè,
Robert Roessle Hospital, Humboldt University at Berlin,
Lindenberger Weg 80, 13122 Berlin, Germany

JOCHAM, D.

Department of Urology, Medical University of Lübeck,
Ratzeburger Allee 160, 23538 Lübeck, Germany

KARPEH, M.S.

Gastric and Mixed Tumor Service, Department of
Surgical Oncology, Memorial Sloan-Kettering Cancer Center,
1275 York Avenue, New York, NY 10021, USA

KOEA, J.B.

Gastric and Mixed Tumor Service, Department
of Surgical Oncology, Memorial Sloan-Kettering Cancer Center,
1275 York Avenue, New York, NY 10021, USA

LABOW, D.M.

Research Fellow, Department of Surgery,
Memorial Sloan-Kettering Cancer center, 1275 York Avenue,
New York, NY 10021, USA

MANN, G.B.

Department of Surgery, Royal Melbourne Hospital,
University of Melbourne, Parkville, 3050, Australia

PAOLUCCI, V.

Department of General and Vascular Surgery
Johann Wolfgang Goethe University
Theodor-Stern Kai 7, 60590 Frankfurt/Main, Germany

RAU, B.

Division of Surgery and Surgical Oncology, University Hospital
Charité, Campus Berlin Buch, Robert-Roessle Hospital
and Tumor Institute, Humboldt University at Berlin,
Lindenberger Weg 80, 13122 Berlin, Germany

Russo, P.
Urology Service, Department of Surgery,
Memorial Sloan-Kettering Cancer Center, 1275 York Avenue,
New York, NY 10021, USA

Schlag, P.M.
Professor and Chairman, Division of Surgery and Surgical
Oncology, University Hospital Charité, Campus Berlin Buch,
Robert-Roessle Hospital and Tumor Institute, Humboldt University at Berlin, Lindenberger Weg 80, 13122 Berlin, Germany

Basic Aspects

Technical Aspects of Pneumoperitoneum and Gasless Laparoscopy

V. Paolucci · C.N. Gutt · W. Bank

Creation of space in the peritoneal cavity was the first condition for successful laparoscopic surgery. With the insufflation of gas, a simple and safe way for sufficient abdominal exposure was found. However, laparoscopy with pneumoperitoneum causes a restriction of the surgeon's freedom of movement. The construction of the laparoscopic instruments is hampered by their small diameter and their length, because its shaft must fit into sealed trocars. Usually these instruments are constructed with an axially located mechanism, which is single or twin action. Every action of a jaw must be transmitted over a central rod in the shaft to a hinge system at the instrument's tip. This leads to reduced tactile sense and restriction of movement for surgeons.

A combination of conventional and laparoscopic surgery under over-pressure conditions is not possible, because the loss of pressure through even a small incision means loss of visualization for the surgeon.

There are also risks in the pneumoperitoneum for the patient.

For these reasons, systems for mechanical distension of the abdominal wall were designed.

Laparoscopy with Pneumoperitoneum

The insufflation of gas into the peritoneum causes the lifting of the abdominal wall that is the necessary condition for laparoscopic exposure and surgery. The intra-abdominal pressure must be constant during the operation, so sealed trocars must be used.

Gas

Today, laparoscopy implies the use of a CO_2 pneumoperitoneum. However, the ideal gas for exposure in the abdominal cavity has not been found. Solubility, diffusibility, combustibility, and possible pharmacological side effects (for example, effects on lung and heart function, infection, as well as tumor growth) are the parameters determining the choice of a gas for use in humans.

Carbon Dioxide

Carbon dioxide (CO_2) is a common product of metabolism. It dissolves very well in the blood fluid physically and chemically. Therefore, the danger of gas embolism is very low. CO_2 does not support combustion, so this gas is commonly used for pneumoperitoneum. However, CO_2 does not behave as an inert element; its reabsorption is modulated by the concentration gradient and by the exposed surface of the microscopic peritoneal vessels, invariably leading to a certain pCO_2 rise both in arterial and venous blood [13]. Under normal conditions a CO_2 extra load increases alveolar ventilation, which brings the $paCO_2$ back to normal levels; during general anesthesia, the gas exchange is dependent upon the mechanically predetermined alveolar ventilation[7]: the CO_2 surplus normally does not exceed 30% of the basal CO_2 load, and consequently a moderate increase in minute ventilation by the same percentage is sufficient to eliminate any excess [10]. The reduction of the basal metabolic rate that is observed during anesthesia is also helpful in decreasing CO_2 production.

Arterial CO_2 rises slowly, and its concentration reaches a continuous level only after 15–30 min. The absorption of CO_2 is directly proportional to the intra-abdominal pressure up to 10–12 mmHg; then, because of the splanchnic vessels and some other factors, a continuous increase in gas reabsorption is not observed [5].

CO_2 removal follows two different pathways. One pathway involves tissue exchange with the venous bloodstream and consequent elimination via the lung; the second pathway is tissue storage in the bones, muscles, and fat [35]. The CO_2 stores of the body may therefore be considered as two compartments with different uptake/elimination rates: the arterial-alveolar store is a high-uptake compartment (max. store 0.15 ml CO_2/kg/mmHg) even with a high elimination rate via ventilation; the slow-uptake compartment behaves as a buffer, storing 0.566 ml/kg/mmHg, up to 120 l of CO_2 [16]. The slow elimination from this compartment causes high CO_2 arterial blood levels postoperatively for a considerable length of time [11].

Arterial CO_2 is reflected by respiratory acidosis with no modification of the base excess, because the H^+ increase is linked to the CO_2 extra load, with no metabolic participation. Such modifications, a slight decrease of the pH value together with normal HCO_3^- and no relevant acid-base imbalance, are not harmful in patients with normal cardiopulmonary function [9]. A relative imbalance may jeopardize patients with relevant heart or lung disease [39].

Room Air

Room air consists of up to 79% nitrogen. In various countries [40] room air is still used for pneumoperitoneum, but it is generally avoided because of its extremely low solubility in blood. Indeed, nitrogen is insoluble in water as well as chemically, and there is some danger of air embolism. Gas remaining in the abdominal cavity will not be absorbed, and it is radiologically visible, as a subphrenic sickle, with the patients having typical complaints.

Oxygen

Plain oxygen (O_2) is a physiological gas, quite tissue compatible, ten times as difficult to absorb as CO_2 gas, and very explosive. Especially when used in cauterization, the formation of hydrogen and explosive gas through electronic splitting has cost some patients and physicians their lives. It was used in the beginning of laparoscopic surgery and has been abandoned as an insufflant for laparoscopy today [14].

Nitrous Oxide

The anesthetic effect of nitrous oxide (N_2O; laughing gas) is well known. For this reason, it has been used mostly in diagnostic upper abdominal laparoscopy under local anesthesia. It is less suitable for operative laparoscopy. On one hand, it dissociates with increasing temperature in N and O_2 (laughing gas danger); on the other hand, it can trigger a large number of undesirable systemic effects. Nitrous oxide, usually considered safe for diagnostic laparoscopy, has been associated with fatal explosions during the use of electrocautery [33]. A recent experimental work [25], however, did not confirm the risk of combustion in the presence of N_2O under normal conditions.

Inert Gases

Helium, xenon, and argon are inert, water-insoluble monoatomic gases. Under pneumoperitoneum conditions with these gases, the troublesome „fogging up" of the scope is not possible – a small advantage because the risk of gas embolism is high. Helium has been suggested as an alternative for pneumoperitoneum because it is not flammable, is nontoxic, and is physiologically inert. It has been used clinically for insufflation [3], and some authors pointed out advantages of pneumoperitoneum with helium relative to CO_2 [32]. Experimental studies proved helium to be dangerous as an agent for gas embolism in the dog. Furthermore, intravascular helium in humans (because of rupture of helium-filled intra-aortic balloon) has been reported to produce neurological deficits, as shown in vascular occlusion by gas bubbles [40]. In addition, the gas is expensive and noneconomical, meaning that it is not commercially available.

Gas Pressure

Under pneumoperitoneum conditions, the potential danger to the patient's safety and the optimal operative exposure have an intricate relationship. Comparing the abdominal cavity with a hemisphere of 30-cm diameter, at a pressure of 12 mmHg/cm^2 the force applied onto the total surface of the parietal peritoneum will reach approximately 33 kp. The abdominal wall will be lifted with a force of approximately 11 kp. The remaining forces will work in equal parts laterally onto the diaphragm, resulting in a further enlargement of the intra-abdominal space, and downward onto the viscera, resulting in a retraction of bowel loops and stomach (Fig. 1). Undesired but unavoidable side effects are reduction of the res-

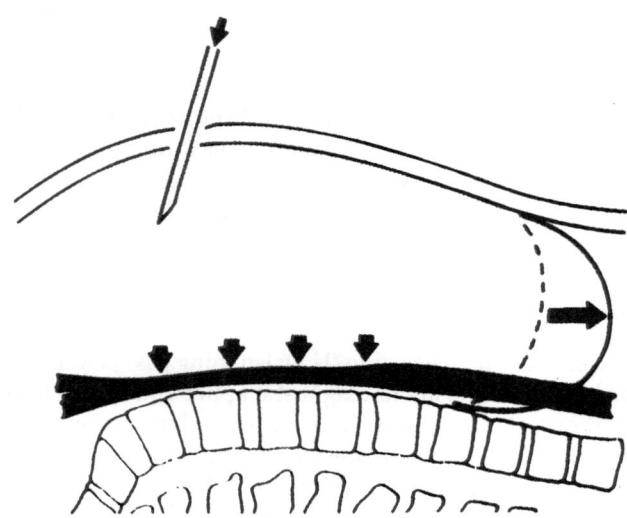

Fig. 1. Consequences of pneumoperitoneum with a pressure of 12 mmHg/cm² on diaphragm and vena cava

piratory minute volume and compression of the vena cava with obstruction of venous blood return to the heart.

These side effects limit the over-pressure in the abdominal cavity to approximately 12 mmHg. This results in a good expansion of the gas bubble. Furthermore, higher pressures rarely lead to an effective enlargement of the gas-filled abdominal cavity, even in obese patients. Whenever the extension reserve of the abdominal muscles is reached, the abdominal wall resistance to additional expansion increases disproportionately, because the intra-abdominal pressure depends on the abdominal muscle tone. Therefore, a complete and constant muscle relaxation is not the only presupposition for optimal intraoperative view; prevention of gas pressure-related complications is also necessary.

The CO₂ Insufflators

The fundamental system for automatic regulation is the monofilar-bivalent-system (MBS). The gas refill stream regulates itself by measuring the actual intra-abdominal pressure through the same opening. The intermittent electronic measurement of the static pressure, meaning the actual intra-abdominal gas pressure (CO_2-PNEU-Electronic), provides consistency of gas bubble size through regulation of the gas refill stream in case of gas loss. Occasionally, it will meet certain limits, though.

In many cases, CO_2 „over-pressure" laparoscopy is the adequate procedure. For patients who are cardially impaired or have hiatal hernias, for example, an intra-abdominal pressure of 12 mmHg may already be too high. In addition, extensive opening of the retroperitoneum, e.g., in parailiac lymph-node dissection, could cause cardiopulmonary problems. Injured small veins, not bleeding because of the over-pressure, could absorb large amounts of gas.

Otherwise, for example, in very obese patients, in patients with intestinal distension, in the case of extensive abdominal adhesions, or when for anesthesiological reasons sufficient muscle relaxation is not possible, a pressure of 12 mmHg is not sufficient. Especially at the lateral borderlines of the gas dome, handling ability is reduced, so efficient operation is not possible.

There can be problems in maintaining the pressure in the abdominal cavity as well. The reason for this could be insufficient sealing of the trocars or the necessity for suction of large amounts of fluid (blood, irrigation liquid) within a short period of time.

Especially during minimally invasive surgery, the upper abdominal cavity collapses very quickly after loss of pressure.

Complications of Laparoscopy with Pneumoperitoneum

Laparoscopy with a pneumoperitoneum causes a restriction of the surgeon's freedom of movement and is the reason for typical complications.

In addition to the physiological consequences of the pneumoperitoneum, there are technical disadvantages. Instruments must be introduced into the abdominal cavity through sealed trocars to maintain the applied intra-abdominal pressure throughout the procedure. This fact adds another difficulty to the construction of these instruments. The construction of these instruments is also hampered by their small diameter and length, because their shaft has to fit into the trocar.

Complications Associated with Insertion of the Veress Needle and the Trocars

Traumatic injuries due to the insertion of the peritoneal needle or to the trocars are described in many studies. The most common complications are associated with improper placement of the insufflation needle: subcutaneous emphysema and pneumoomentum occur frequently, but in general are not serious. In 1990, Albert Yuzpe [41] carried out a mailing survey regarding laparoscopic procedures. Among 407 physicians asked about pneumoperitoneum needle and trocar injuries, more than one-quarter reported some injury related either to the primary or secondary trocar or to the pneumoperitoneum needle; 16.7% of physicians reported organ injuries (bladder, bowel, or vessels) caused by the pneumoperitoneum needle (Veress needle); 16.5% ascribed major injuries to the primary trocar and 9.1% to the secondary trocar.

Injuries caused by the Veress needle are not often problematic, whereas injuries caused by trocars must be corrected by laparoscopic or open surgery. Perforations of the gastrointestinal tract are generally quickly recognized and accessible to immediate repair. Liver and spleen injuries have also been described. Table 1 gives an overview of the incidence of various organ injuries.

Table 1. Complications associated with insertion of the laparoscope

Complication	Incidence (%)	Authors
Abdominal wall bleeding	0.03	Henning and Look 1985 [23]
Urinary tract injury	0.02	Brown 1978 [4]
GI tract perforation<?1>	0.08	Henning and Look 1985 [23]]
	0.18	Brown 1978 [4]
Liver, spleen injury	0.04	Henning and Look 1985 [23]
Omental injury	0.10	Henning and Look 1985 [23]
Pelvic side wall or ovarian vessel injury	0.09	Brown 1978 [4]

Complications Associated with Gas Insufflation

CO_2 pneumoperitoneum results in a significant transperitoneal absorption, with secondary hypercapnia and acidemia. The accumulation of CO_2 is also associated with an increase in systemic and pulmonary arterial pressure. The heart rate increases to compensate for the decreased stroke volume to maintain cardiac output [24].

The induction and maintenance of a pneumoperitoneum are associated with adverse cardiovascular, respiratory, and metabolic changes, which could end in complications like bradyarrhythmia (during CO_2 insufflation) [29] or asystolic cardiac arrest due probably to a fatal CO_2 embolism [37]. A sequence of 54 cardiorespiratory accidents during insufflation of the peritoneum shows that there is a risk [28].

Tension pneumothorax has also been described in patients with diaphragm injuries. However, most of the hemodynamic changes are due to the pressure in the peritoneal cavity rather than to CO_2 gas absorption, because the complications are similar under pneumoperitoneum produced by other gases [15].

Table 2 gives an overview of the incidence of complications associated with the pneumoperitoneum.

Complications After Laparoscopy

Wound complications occur quite often. One of these complications is hematoma, usually secondary to injuries of the abdominal wall vessel when the trocars are inserted; another complication is wound infection by contamination from an infected gallbladder or calculi. Prolonged pain after the operation is unusual and may represent a complication such as hematoma (Table 3).

Table 2. Complications associated with the pneumoperitoneum

Complication	Incidence (%)	Authors
Pneumothorax	0.01	Henning and Look 1985 [23]
Arrhythmia	0.01	Henning and Look 1985 [23]
	47.0	Myles 1991 [29]
	41.5	Phillips and Keith 1975 [31]
Bradyarrhythmia	30.0	Myles 1991 [29]
Cardiac arrest	0.041	Shifren et al. 1992 [37]
	5.0	Phillips and Keith 1975 [31]
Air embolus	1.7	Phillips and Keith 1975 [31]
Subcutaneous emphysema	0.26	Henning and Look 1985 [23]
Vasovagal hypotension	0.14	Henning and Look 1985 [23]
Mediastinal emphysema	0.03	Henning and Look 1985 [23]

Table 3. Postlaparoscopy complications

Complication	Incidence (%)	Authors
Prolonged pain	0.04	Henning and Look 1985 [23]
Hernia at insertion site	0.01	Henning and Look 1985 [23]
Infection	0.20	Collet et al. 1993 [8]
Hematoma	0.50	Collet et al. 1993 [8]

Laparoscopic Surgery Without Pneumoperitoneum

The use of laparoscopic methods in surgery depends essentially on the establishment of an intraperitoneal space that allows a good exposure of the organ of interest. For this purpose, insufflation of CO_2 gas has routinely been used for extension of the abdominal wall. Laparoscopy with a pneumoperitoneum causes a restriction of the instrument's freedom of movement and can be the reason for typical complications.

In addition to physiological consequences of the pneumoperitoneum, there are technical disadvantages. Instruments must be introduced into the abdominal cavity through sealed trocars to maintain the applied intra-abdominal pressure throughout the procedure. This adds another difficulty to the construction of these instruments. The construction of these instruments is hampered by their small diameter and length, because their shaft has to be circular and must fit into the trocar. In laparoscopy without pneumoperitoneum conventional instruments for open surgery and simple rubber trocars can be used because sealing is not necessary in the absence of intra-abdominal pressure. In addition, it is possible to use instruments without laparoscopic equivalents, which could not be designed to fit through sealed trocars [19, 21].

Thus alternative methods for mechanical distension of the abdominal wall have been explored. The following retraction systems are developed to provide exposure for adequate visualization of the viscera in combination with a low-pressure pneumoperitoneum or even completely without a pneumoperitoneum. Mechanical distension of the abdominal cavity is achieved with intra-abdominal and subcutaneous lifting. Two intra-abdominal systems combine traction of the abdominal wall with pressure on the internal organs. Every system allows the use of all laparoscopic instruments originally designed for pneumoperitoneum. Only in the absence of a pneumoperitoneum can conventional instruments be used.

Intra-abdominal Retraction Systems

Abdominal Cavity Expander-System ACE-WISAP (Semm), T-Shaped Endoscopic Retractor (Gazayerli), and Sling (Banting and Cuschieri)

Method: Point lifting
Requirements: Permanent low-pressure pneumoperitoneum
Materials: Reusable steel

The *abdominal cavity expander* [36] is a T-shaped retractor that helps to maintain the volume inside the abdominal cavity, for example, in the case of loss of gas during laparoscopy with pneumoperitoneum. It can be introduced through a 5-mm as well as a 10-mm port and will avoid the need to convert to laparotomy. A similar *T-shaped* fan described by Gazayerli [18] is used to provide an isolated area of lift for additional exposure during laparoscopy with pneumoperitoneum. The *sling* [2] retracts the upper abdominal wall and the falciform ligament together and consists of a flexible plastic tube. The two ends of the tube are tied together and attached to a frame work above the operating table. Tube placement is achieved with a metal introducer.

Winch Retractor (Araki), U-Shaped Retractor (Kitano), Coathanger (Maher)

Method: Linear lifting
Requirements: Initial pneumoperitoneum
Materials: Reusable steel

The *winch retractor* [1] consists of a curved Kirschner wire attached to the adjustable chain of two table-based winches. The wire is inserted percutaneously through all layers of the abdominal wall into the peritoneal cavity. During laparoscopic cholecystectomy the pneumoperitoneum is decompressed after the gallbladder is retracted by grasping the fundus. The *U-shaped retractor* [26] is introduced into the abdominal cavity with a guide tube under endoscopic control after initial installation of a pneumoperitoneum. A frame work and winches provide abdominal wall retraction. After pneumoperitoneum the *coathanger*-shaped retractor is inserted into the abdominal cavity through an incision lateral to the epigastric vessels and exits lateral to the epigastric vessels at the other side of the abdomen. The retractor is fixed to a chain by which it is elevated.

Pelvi-Snake (Volz) and Suspendor 3-X (Mouret)

Method: Planar lifting
Requirements: Initial pneumoperitoneum
Materials: Reusable steel

The *Pelvi-Snake* [38] consists of a steel spring that is screwed into the abdomen 5 cm below the umbilicus through a 3-mm incision. With a diameter of 15 cm, it covers an area of approximately 150 cm² inside the abdomen. A simple metal rod that easily rests loosely on a table-fixed frame is responsible for clamping the Pelvi-Snake. Via mini-laparotomy the *Suspendor 3-X* [17], a gallows-shaped metal bar, is inserted for additional security after a pneumoperitoneum is built up. The base is fastened laterally to the table. A screw system allows regulation of the tent-shaped abdominal wall elevation.

Peritoneal Cavity Augmentation PCA (Schaller)

Method: Linear lifting
Requirements: Initial pneumoperitoneum, permanent low-pressure
               pneumoperitoneum
Materials: Reusable steel, reusable pressure body

Peritoneal cavity augmentation [34] applies traction to the abdominal wall and, at the same time, mechanical pressure on internal organs. Two sleeves are introduced percutaneously near the operational field under endoscopic control. An internal connector is attached under light compression of the abdominal wall. At the tips of two metal rods, which are conducted in the sleeves, a flat translucent pressure body is coupled and placed on the internal organs under view. A suspension at the operating table allows lifting of the abdominal wall.

Spreading Trocars (Dragojevic)

Method: Point lifting
Requirements: Initial air insufflation
Materials: Reusable steel

After initial air insufflation a safety trocar is placed. After abdominal inspection the safety trocar is substituted by a trocar with a spreading device [12]. When a reduction socket is introduced into the trocar, the split tip is pushed outward and a stable fixture in the abdominal wall emerges. After the first trocar is attached to a gallows, additional spreading trocars are placed and suspended. The desired pulling force can be applied separately (Fig. 2).

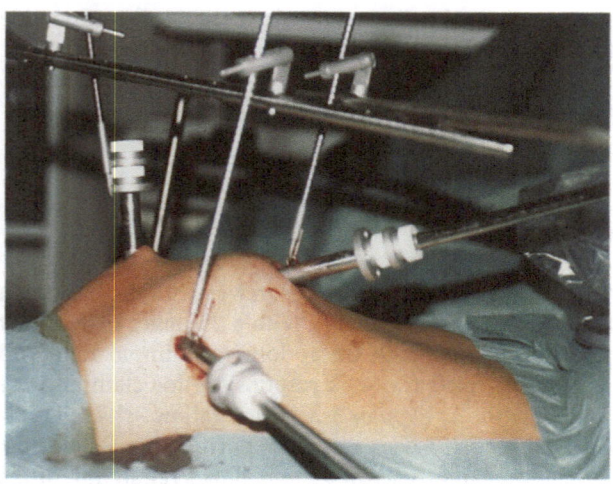

Fig. 2. Outside picture of laparoscopy with hanging spreading trocars (Dragojevic)

Laparolift (Chin)

Method:	Planar lifting
Requirements:	Isopneumic conditions
Materials:	Disposable plastic/metal fan

The *Laparolift* [6] contains a special retraction device made of high-strength plastic with two blades, which is introduced through a 2-cm incision into the abdominal cavity and fanned to conform to the abdominal wall. This retraction device (Laparofan) is attached to the tip of an electric-powered lift arm, which raises and lowers with the push of a button. In addition to the Laparofan, the laparoscope is introduced through the same incision.

Vario Lift Retraction System (Gutt)

Method:	Planar lifting
Requirements:	Isopneumic conditions
Materials:	Reusable steel

The *Vario Lift Retraction System* [20] is introduced via a 2-cm mini-laparotomy. For abdominal wall retraction two lifting parts of different size and shape are assembled to create a intraperitoneal frame. With combinations of these parts the retractor can be adjusted to different abdominal quadrants and the patient's individual anatomy. After a correct positioning under endoscopic control it is attached to an outside mechanical lifting arm that is suspended over the operating table (Fig. 3). According to the needs for visualization a translucent plastic membrane can be unfolded and placed for posterior organ retraction using the same access.

Fig. 3a–c. The Vario Lift Retraction System (Gutt). a The lifting arm is fixed at the operating table. b The lifting parts are placed through a 2-cm laparotomy. c The abdominal wall is lifted

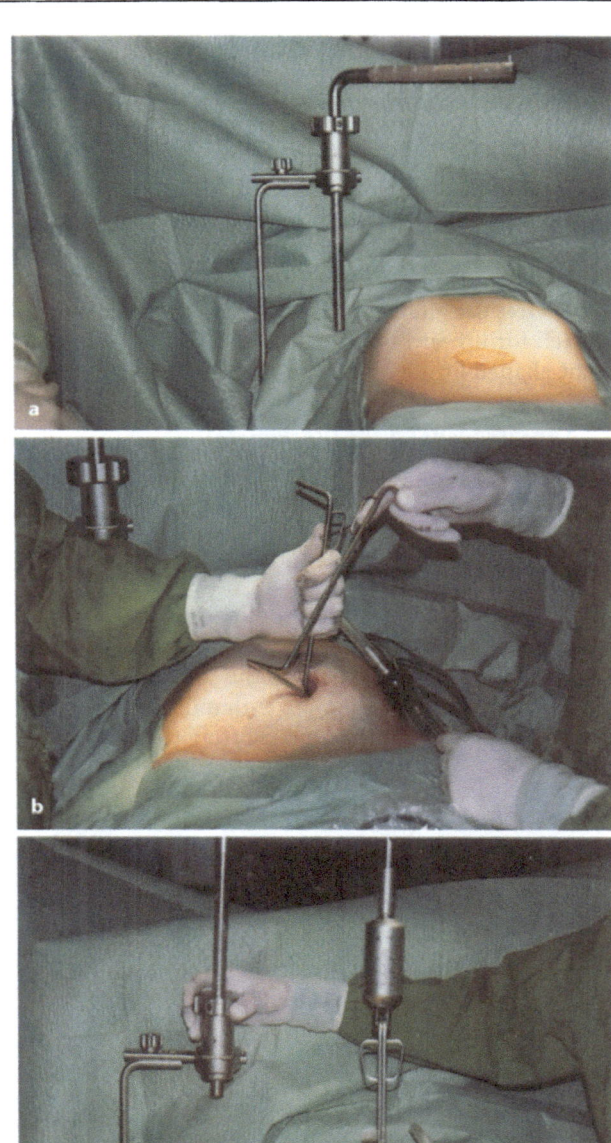

Subcutaneous Retraction Systems

Tent-Shaped Wiring (Nagai)

Method: Linear lifting
Requirements: Isopneumic conditions
Materials: Reusable steel

The system consists of two wire loops that anchor subcutaneously in the skin. The wires are attached to lifting handles, and a winching device is tightened and raised for upward traction. The raising of the wire loops produces single-point, tent-shaped lifting of the skin in two places [30].

Subcutaneous Wiring (Hashimoto)

Method: Linear/planar lifting
Requirements: Isopneumic conditions
Materials: Reusable steel

Subcutaneous wires with a defined shape are tunneled and suspended with winches to a Kent retractor to achieve abdominal wall lifting. Sutures are used on both sides as hangers to lift up the subcutaneous wires. If the lifting effect is not satisfactory a thin metal plate with multiple holes is placed between the subcutaneous wires for better-balanced lifting (Fig. 4) [22].

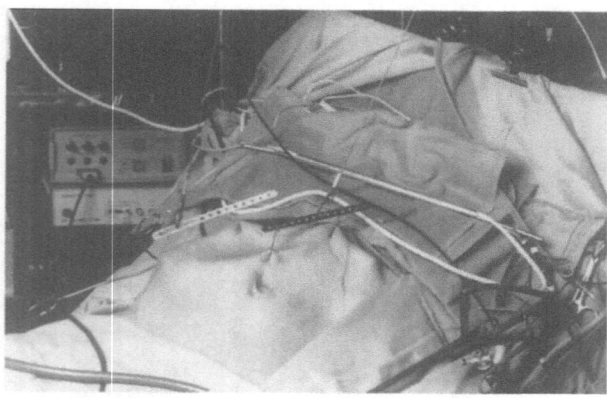

Fig. 4. Final setup in abdominal lifting with subcutaneous wiring and adjustable plate lifting (Hashimoto)

Laparo Tenser (Lucini)

Method: Planar lifting
Requirements: Isopneumic conditions
Materials: Reusable steel

The system consists of an abdominal wall retractor with two convex-shaped sub-cutaneous needles that can be attached to a mechanical lifting arm. To improve exposure, low-pressure CO_2 insufflation can be added.

Effective retraction systems work under isopneumic conditions. Nevertheless, some systems require an additional permanent low-pressure pneumoperitoneum because the extent of intra-abdominal exposure is not sufficient (T-shaped endoscopic retractor [18] and sling [2], ACE-WISAP [36], peritoneal cavity augmentation, PCA [37]). Laparoscopy with mechanical wall lifting in combination with a low-pressure pneumoperitoneum differs from conventional laparoscopy with a pneumoperitoneum only in the technique by which an intra-abdominal space for adequate vision of the viscera is achieved. The expense of the installation of a pneumoperitoneum is increased by the additional system setup for mechanical retraction. This may help to prevent typical complications and provide additional exposure in isolated areas during laparoscopy with reduced gas insufflation, but there are no technical advantages with regard to instrumentation. The instruments still must be introduced through sealed trocars to maintain the intra-abdominal pressure. The construction of these instruments is hampered by their small diameter and length, because their shaft must fit into the trocars. Tactile sensitivity of the surgeon using laparoscopic instruments with a hinge system or hingeless instruments is reduced to a great extent, because of their axially located mechanism with the in-and-out movement of a central rod. The action of the jaw must be transmitted either by two hinge systems or by a hingeless system with outside-bent jaws. The actions of both instrument designs have high friction and reduced force feedback. In combination with a low-pressure pneumoperitoneum only laparoscopic instruments are useful.

Several intra-abdominal systems require an initial pneumoperitoneum for a safe introduction of intra-abdominal retraction devices under endoscopic guidance (winch retractor [1], U-shaped retractor [26], Suspendor 3-X [17]). These techniques do not minimize the risk of needle injuries. After system setup the pneumoperitoneum is decompressed. Abdominal wall lifting mostly creates in these systems a more tent-shaped suspension with limited intra-abdominal exposure. The Pelvi-Snake [38] creates a more dome-shaped suspension, but its application is limited to the pelvic region. Besides optic and instrument ports, these systems require additional access for mechanical retraction. Conventional surgical techniques can be applied after system setup. Spreading trocars [12] combine intraperitoneal access with lifting of the abdominal wall, but there is no technical advantage with regard to instrumentation. The peritoneal cavity augmentation system [34] combines a low-pressure pneumoperitoneum with abdominal wall traction and mechanical pressure to internal organs and provides a good exposure. Procedures without specimen removal can be performed with small laparoscopic instruments under local anesthesia. The concept of this retraction system focuses on a further reduction of invasiveness in combination with gas insufflation.

Laparoscopy completely without pneumoperitoneum eliminates the hindrance of intra-abdominal pressure and gastightness. Intra-abdominal systems, the disposable fan-shaped retractor [6] and the Vario Lift Retraction System [20], are inserted under direct digital guidance together with the optic trocar through a small incision. Additional access for system setup is not required. Both systems provide a planar suspension of the abdominal wall; however, the intraperitoneal frame of the Vario Lift Retraction System creates a better lateral exposure and a more dome-shaped suspension without tenting effects. The combination of its lifting parts provides individual adjustment for the patient's anatomy and creates a retractor shape for every abdominal region. Compared with a pneumoperitoneum the Vario Lift Retraction System [20] allows application of mechanical pressure on internal organs. According to the need for visualization a translucent plastic membrane can be unfold and placed for posterior organ retraction. The disposable fan retractor [6] is available in different designs for each abdominal quadrant.

Subcutaneous retraction systems do not require initial pneumoperitoneum; however, to improve exposure CO_2 insufflation can be added simply. Otherwise, in the absence of pneumoperitoneum conventional instruments can be used. System setup of subcutaneous wiring [22] is more complicated in comparison to the Laparo Tenser.

When only intra-abdominal exposure is considered, no mechanical retraction system can compete with a CO_2 pneumoperitoneum. The advantage is that, in combination with microsurgical laparoscopic instruments, limited procedures without specimen removal may be performed under local anesthesia. On the other hand, if a slightly limited exposure to the region of interest is acceptable in the absence of intraperitoneal insufflation, surgical qualities that originally were lost with the establishment of laparoscopic techniques are regained. From a practical standpoint the surgeon is allowed to combine the advantages of endoscopic surgery, such as magnified videoendoscopic visualization, with well-known open surgical techniques to create a symbiosis of proven methods. For example, the use of conventional ring forceps, lap sponges, and insulated, bended right angles increases the radius of manipulation and improves the exposure, for example, of the gallbladder and the triangle of Calot. Preparation of fine structures and tissue with the surgeon's experienced sense of touch is more efficient. Instead of time-consuming knot tying techniques and expensive staplers, extracorporal knot tying has proved to be a fast and easy procedure. The surgeon's finger palpating tissue and organ surfaces is the most sensitive instrument. In laparoscopy under isopneumic conditions there is no hindrance to direct touch of the surgeon's hand. Careful specimen removal is facilitated by using conventional forceps under constant laparoscopic control. Differences between laparoscopy and open surgery can be overcome. The shorter operating time and limited technical expenditure are cost-efficient.

■ References

1. Araki K, Namikawa K, Yamamoto H, Mizutani J,Doiguchi M, Arai M, Yamaguchi T, Uno K, Ido Y, Hayashi N, Ogawa M (1993) Abdominal wall retraction during laparoscopic cholecystectomy. World J Surg 17:105–108
2. Banting S, Shimi S, van der Velpen G, Cuschieri A (1993) Abdominal wall lifting: low-pressure pneumoperitoneum laparoscopic surgery. Surg Endosc 7:57–59
3. Bongard FS, Pianim N, Liu SY (1991) Using helium for insufflation during laparoscopy. JAMA 266:3131
4. Brown CG (1978) Gynaecological laparoscopy: report on the confidential enquiry into gynaecological laparoscopy. London: Royal College of Obstetricians and Gynaecologists 1978
5. Cherniack NS, Longobardo GS, Staw I, Heymann M (1966) Dynamics of carbon dioxide stores changes following an alteration in ventilation. J Appl Physiol 21:785–793
6. Chin AK, Moll FH, McColl MB, et al (1993) Mechanical peritoneal retraction as a replacement for carbon dioxide pneumoperitoneum. J Am Assoc Gynecol Laparosc 1:62–66
7. Ciofolo MJ, Clergue F, Seebacher J, Lefebvre G, Viars P (1990) Ventilatory effects of laparoscopy under epidural anesthesia. Anesth Analg 70:357–361
8. Collet D, Edye M, Perissat J (1993) Conversions and complications of laparoscopic cholecystectomy. Surg Endosc 7:334–338
9. De Cosmo G, Primieri P, Gualtieri E, Bonomo V, Grottola A, Villani A (1992) Modificazioni respiratorie in corso di colecistectomia per via laparoscopica. Min Anest 58:825–826
10. De Sousa H, Tyler IL (1987) Can absorption of the insufflation gas during laparoscopy be hazardous? Anesthesiology 67:A476
11. Deyo GA (1992) Complications of laparoscopic cholecystectomy. Surg Laparosc Endosc 2:41–48
12. Dragojevic B, Tomic D (1996) Multifunctional trocars as suspension devices for gas-free laparoscopic operations. Min Invas Ther Allied Technol 5:95–98
13. Dureuil B.(1994) Modifications peroperatoites de la fonction respiratoire. Edition Techniques, Encyl Med Chir, Paris, Anesthesie-Reanimation, 36–374 B–10, 7
14. Fevers C (1933) Die Laparoskopie mit dem Cystoskop. Med Klinik 31:1042–1045
15. Fitzgerald SD, Andrus CH, Baudendistel LJ (1992) Hypercarbia during carbon dioxide pneumoperitoneum. Am J Surg 163:186–190
16 Fowle AS, Campbell EJM (1964) The immediate carbon dioxide storage capacity of man. Clin Sci 27:41–46
17. Francois Y, Mouret P (1992) Suspenseur de paroi et coelio-chirurgie. J Chir129:492–493
18. Gazayerli MM (1991) The Gazayerli endoscopic retractor model 1. Surg Laparosc Endosc 1:98–100
19. Gutt CN, Held S, Voepel H, Paolucci V (1996) Instruments for gasless laparoscopic surgery. Min Invas Ther Allied Technol 5:307–312
20. Gutt CN, Heinz P, Held S, Paolucci V, Encke A (1996) Modular retraction system (MORES) for gasless laparoscopy. Surg Endosc 10:584
21. Gutt CN, Voepel H, Linker R, Bamberg W (1996) Conventional surgical instruments for gasless laparoscopy. In: Paolucci V, Schaeff B (eds) Gasless laparoscopy in general surgery and gynecology. Thieme, Stuttgart, New York, pp 138–144
22. Hashimoto D, Nayeem SA, Kajiwara S, Hoshino T (1993) Laparoscopic cholecystectomy: an approach without pneumoperitoneum. Surg Endosc 7:54–56
23. Henning H, Look D (1985) Laparoskopie Atlas und Lehrbuch. Thieme, Stuttgart
24. Ho HS, Gunther RA, Wolfe BM (1992) Intraperitoneal carbon dioxide insufflation and cardiopulmonary functions. Arch Surg 127:928–933

25. Hunter JG, Staheli J, Oddsdottir M, Trus T (1995) Nitrous oxide pneumoperitoneum revisited. Is there a risk of combustion? Surg Endosc 9:501–504
26. Kitano S, Iso Y, Tomikawa M, Moriyama M, Sugimachi K (1993) A prospective randomized trial comparing pneumoperitoneum and u-shaped retractor elevation for laparoscopic cholecystectomy. Surg Endosc 7:311–314
27. Melzer A, Buess G, Cuschieri A (1992) Instruments for endoscopic surgery. In: Cuschieri A, Buess G, Perissat J (eds) Operative manual of endoscopic surgery. Springer, Berlin Heidelberg, pp 14–36
28. Mintz M (1977) Risks and prophylaxis in laparoscopy: a survey of 100,000 cases. J Reprod Med 18:269–272
29. Myles PS (1991) Bradyarrhythmias and laparoscopy: a prospective study of heart rate changes with laparoscopy. J Obstet Gynaccol 31:171–178
30. Nagai H, Konodo Y, Yasuda T, Kasahara K, Kanazawa K (1993) An abdominal wall-lift method of laparoscopic cholecystectomy without pneumoperitoneal insufflation. Surg Laparos Endos 3:175–179
31. Phillips J, Keith D (1976) Gynecologic laparoscopy in 1975. J Reprod Med 16:105–116
32. Rademaker BMP, Bannenberg JJG, Kalkman CJ, Meyer DW (1995) Effects of pneumoperitoneum with helium on hemodynamics and oxygen transport: a comparison with carbon dioxide. J Laparoendosc Surg 5:15–20
33. Robinson JS, Thompson JM, Wood AW (1979) Fire and explosion hazards in operating theatres: a reply and new evidence. Br J Anaesth 51:90
34. Schaller G, Engelke V, Manegold BC (1996) Mechanical augmentation of the peritoneal cavity in laparoscopic surgery – a new instrument set. Min Invas Ther Allied Technol 5:21–24
35. Seed RF, Shakespeare TF, Muldoon MJ (1970) Carbon dioxide homeostasis during anesthesia for laparoscopy. Anaesthesia 25:223–231
36. Semm K, Lehmann-Willenbrock (1996) Pelvioscopy and laparoscopy without over-pressure – the aspiration pneumoperitoneum. In: Paolucci V, Schaeff B (eds) Gasless laparoscopy in general surgery and gynecology. Thieme, Stuttgart, New York, pp 29–33
37. Shifren JL, Adlestein L, Finkler NJ (1992) Asystolic cardiac arrest: a rare complication of laparoscopy. J Obstet Gynaecol 5:840–841
38. Volz J, Köster S, Weiß M (1996) Developments in gasless gynecologic pelioscopy. In: Paolucci V, Schaeff B (eds) Gasless laparoscopy in general surgery and gynecology. Thieme, Stuttgart New York, pp 108–114
39. Weyland W, Crozier TA, Braun U (1993) Anästesiologische Besonderheiten der operativen Phase bei laparoskopischen Operationen. Zentralbl Chir 118:582–587
40. Wolf JS, Carrier S, Stoller ML (1994) Gas embolism: helium is more lethal than carbon dioxide. J Laparoendosc Surg 4:173–177
41. Yuzpe A (1990) Pneumoperitoneum needle and trocar injuries in laparoscopy. J Reprod Med 35:485–490

Equipment and Strategies of Staging Laparoscopy

D.M. Labow · K.C. Conlon

Historical Perspective

The tenth century Arabian physician Abulkasim (936–1013) [1] is credited with the first documented use of reflected light to view an internal body cavity. Although the procedure was successful, thermal injury from the light source limited the technique. Improvements in optics in the latter half of the nineteenth century rekindled interest in the procedure. Around the turn of the nineteenth century, in Europe, particularly in Austria and Germany, many different centers were exploring endoscopy and laparoscopy. Kussmaul used a primitive endoscope to inspect the stomach of a professional sword swallower and later, in 1869, Karl Stoerk, an Austrian laryngologist, inspected the esophagus of a patient with an instrument comprised of different jointed segments that could be straightened after insertion. In 1901, Georg Kelling [2], a German physician, coined the term „celioscopy" in describing his use of a cystoscope to examine the peritoneal cavity of a dog, utilizing insufflation with air. In 1910, Jacobaeus [3], a Swedish physician, reported the first use of celioscopy in humans and in 1912 he published a 97-patient series [4]. The first reported use of laparoscopy in the United States occurred in 1911 when Bertram Bernheim of Johns Hopkins University performed „organoscopy" on two patients [5], one of which was a patient of W.S. Halstead, diagnosing localized pancreatic cancer, which was later confirmed at open laparotomy by Dr. Halstead.

Heinz Kalk built upon the work of Jacobeus and, in fact, opened a school for laparoscopy in Germany in the 1920s. He made a number of key advances including the introduction of the angled telescope as well as describing a multiport procedure for performing liver biopsies. The next major advance was made by Veress in 1938 with the development of a needle that was inserted into the abdominal cavity to induce pneumoperitoneum. Over the next 40 years, a number of surgeons contributed to the refinement of laparoscopy by varying the number of ports as well as the placement of the laparoscope. However, the use of laparoscopy remained outside the mainstream of clinical practice. It could be argued that it was the work of Kurt Semm, a gynecologist who introduced the automatic insufflator in the 1970s, that ushered in the modern era of laparoscopy [6]. The ability to automatically regulate gas flow and abdominal pressure significantly reduced the incidence of bowel perforations as well as injury to other intra-abdominal and retroperitoneal structures [7]. Semm's contributions did not end with the automatic insufflator. He developed a thermocoagulator to help reduce the injuries caused by unipolar cautery. He also developed the angled-lens scope and hook scissors to allow better visualization and manipulation of pelvic structures. With Hasson's development of the „open" technique of cannula insertion in the late 1970s [8], laparoscopy became a safe and effective procedure with innumerable applications. In fact, by 1984, Semm had performed over 14,000 laparoscopic procedures with an overall complication rate of 0.28% [9]. Despite these advances, it was not until the introduction of the laparoscopic cholecystectomy, which was first performed in 1988 independently by Mouret [10] in France and McKernan and Saye [11] in the United States that laparoscopic surgery gained widespread acceptance.

Over the past decade, the use of laparoscopy has expanded into virtually every surgical discipline, with surgical oncology being no exception. In fact, much of the early work of Jacobeus in 1910 focused on the diagnosis of malignant disease. Today, with the many advancements and refinements that have taken place, there has been a revival in the use of laparoscopy in the diagnosis and staging of malignant disease.

Setup and Equipment

As with any surgical procedure, an appropriate setup of the operating room is critical for efficient, safe, and effective diagnostic laparoscopy.

For most procedures the patient is placed supine on the operating table with the surgeon positioned on the right side. The assistant and/or camera operator stands on the opposite side of the patient. It is our preference for the monitors to be placed above the operative field (Fig. 1). However, alternate monitor positions such as below the level of the operating table may also be used.

Laparoscopic instrumentation is being developed at such a rapid rate that it is virtually impossible to discuss all the tools available to the surgeon today. There is, however, a basic set of equipment necessary for safe and effective diagnostic laparoscopy. Considerable controversy exists as to whether disposable, reusable, or combination disposable–reusable instrumentation is preferable. This discussion is outside the scope of this chapter. However, it should be stated that individual instrument choices should be based on surgeon preference, cost, and availability. At Memorial Sloan-Kettering Cancer Center we utilize a reusable basic set-up. Standard instruments are shown in Fig. 2. The basic tray consists of a scissors, a grasper, and a dissector. Reusable ports are also used (Fig. 3) as well as a partially reusable suction irrigation device. Because electrocautery is used during the procedure, all instruments are insulated to the tip. This setup fulfills our needs as well as being extremely cost-effective. Introducing such a basic setup has contributed to an 80% reduction in the unit cost of a laparoscopic procedure at our institution.

Laparoscopic telescopes are either forward viewing (0°) or oblique (30°–45°). Oblique views are essential to visualize relatively inaccessible regions of the abdomen such as the dome of the liver. In our opinion, the oblique telescope is an essential part of diagnostic laparoscopy in that a full view of the entire abdomen is vital for an accurate staging procedure. The telescope has an eyepiece at the

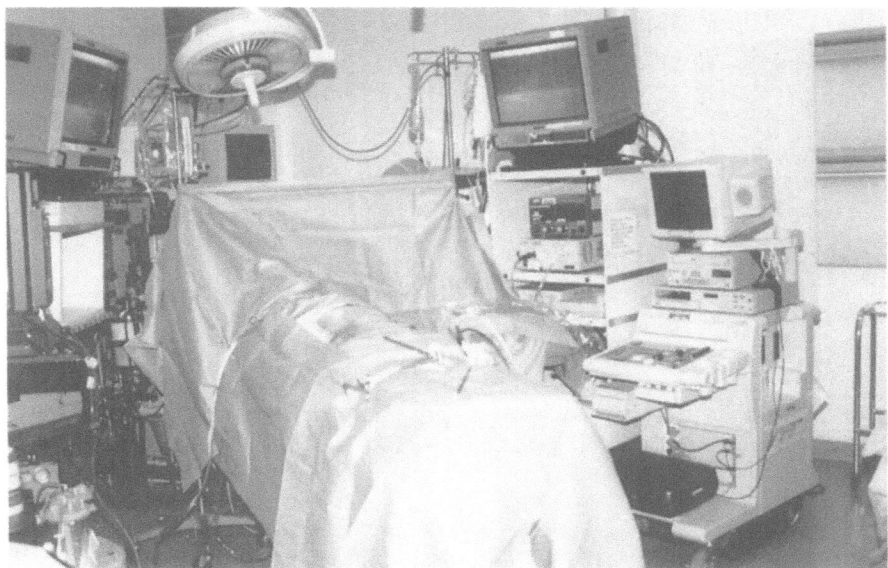

Fig. 1. Operative setup

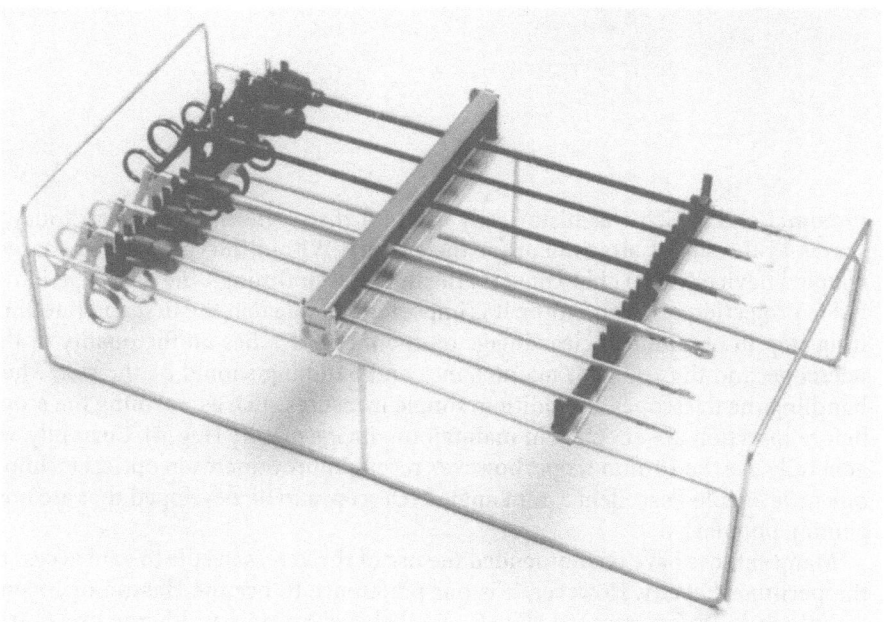

Fig. 2. Standard instrument tray

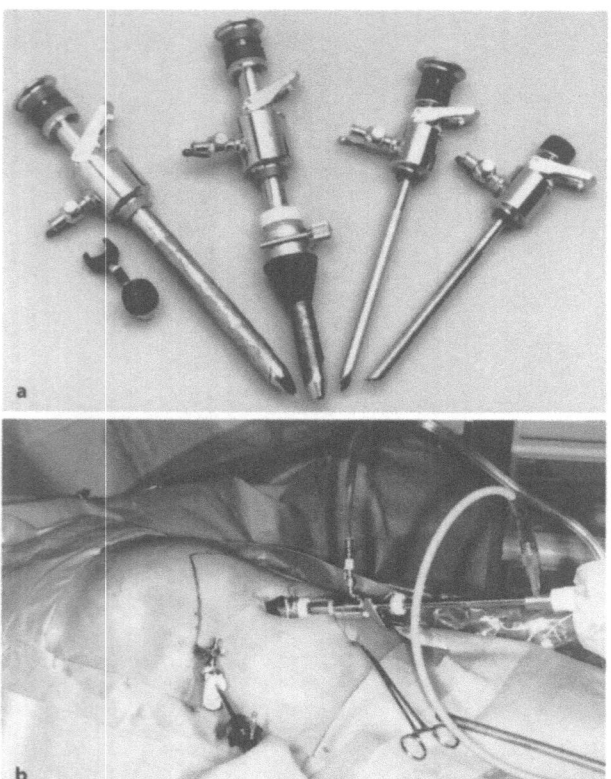

Fig.3. a Reusable laparoscopic trocars.
b Placement of ports in periumbilical area and along the line of proposed open incision

proximal end, which was historically used for direct viewing, although today it serves as the site of attachment for the camera. Within the camera, the charge-coupled device (CCD) chip converts the image seen through the telescope into a video projection on the monitor. It is important to note that the first and rate-limiting step in obtaining a clear image on the monitor relies on the quality of the telescope, and thus diligent maintenance and handling should be the rule when handling the telescopes. In addition, simple measures such as warming the scope before insertion are effective in maintaining image quality (Fig. 4). Currently, we generally use the 10-mm scope; however, recent improvements in optical technology have enabled excellent 5-mm angled telescopes to be developed that are now gaining popularity.

Many authors have recommended the use of the Veress needle to gain access to the peritoneal cavity. However, it is our preference to use the Hasson or „open" technique for safety reasons (Fig. 5). We believe that this technique greatly reduces the risk of bowel or vascular injury seen with the Veress needle, particularly in patients who have had previous surgery. Once access to the abdomen is secured, the telescope is inserted through the umbilical port. After the entire ab-

Fig.4. Thermos flask used for warming telescope before insertion into the abdominal
cavity

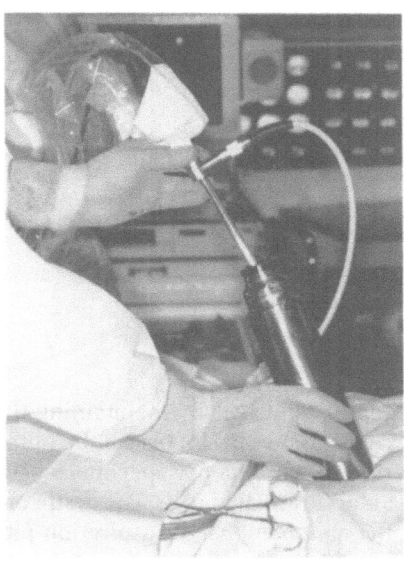

Fig.5. Open technique for
open insertion of initial
trocar. Periumbilical area
is ordinarily preferred;
however, previous situa-
tion may dictate another
site for initial placement

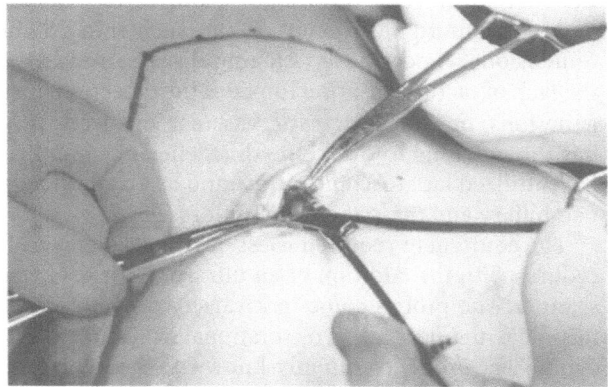

domen and pelvis are surveyed, some dissection and manipulation is usually necessary to gain access to all structures. It is important to emphasize that all dissection should be performed under direct vision.

Once the dissection is complete and the surgeon has access to all intra-abdominal structures, he or she can proceed with the staging procedure. In essence, the
laparoscopic staging should mimic the procedure performed at open operation.
The ability to obtain tissue safely for pathological evaluation is important. Both
cup and grasping forceps are effective instruments, achieving an adequate specimen for pathological evaluation (Fig. 6). Cup forceps help reduce the amount of

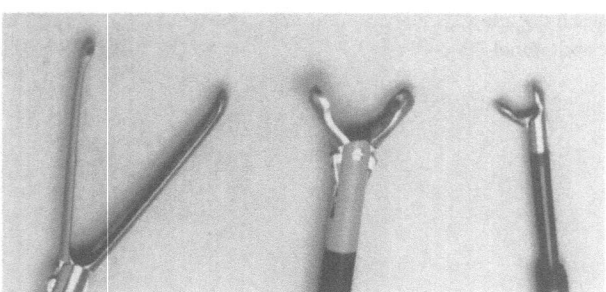

Fig. 6. Biopsy instruments

tumor „spillage" by maintaining the entire specimen within the jaws of the forceps. Tissue specimens can be obtained using a variety of techniques. For larger tumors, core biopsy specimens usually provide the best possibility of obtaining an accurate diagnosis. For cystic or fluid-filled lesions as well as for free fluid in the abdomen, needle aspiration provides an alternative method to obtain cytological specimens. Brush cytology is also effective for lesions not amenable to core biopsy or needle aspiration.

As the prevalence of minimal-access surgery for staging purposes increases, new equipment and techniques continue to emerge. Laparoscopic ultrasound and ultrasound-guided biopsy is one such entity. Standard laparoscopy is a two-dimensional modality. For staging diseases such as peripancreatic malignancy the lack of tactile sensation impedes the detection of small intraparenchymal liver lesions, or retropancreatic vascular involvement. Intraoperative ultrasound has the potential to overcome this deficiency [12–14]. At Memorial Hospital we have utilized laparoscopic ultrasound as an adjunct in the staging of gastric, hepatobiliary and peripancreatic tumors (Fig. 3).

The equipment required is essentially the same as for other laparoscopic procedures with the addition of an ultrasound transducer probe and an ultrasound scanner. The probes come in a variety of configurations, rigid, 2-way or 4-way flexible with linear array, or rotational transducers. There is also a front-viewing, cylindrical probe, commonly known as a sector probe, which is best used for small structures deep in the operative field. Most probes have a Doppler feature, which enhances the information provided to the surgeon regarding the proximity of blood vessels or the bile duct to the area under investigation.

The technique of laparoscopic ultrasound should be organized and meticulous, following the same principles of conventional ultrasound. The transducer probe is passed over the organ under examination in a standard, organized fashion to ensure consistent results. Any abnormality found should be confirmed in two planes to rule out artifact. After a relatively short learning curve for the surgeon, laparoscopic ultrasound is an effective, reproducible test that adds little time to the operation and is cost-effective.

Radioimmuno-guided biopsy is an innovative procedure that is being examined for use for laparoscopic staging procedures [15, 16]. Its use has evolved from recent experience with breast and malignant melanoma. Radioactive colloid alone or in combination with dye is injected around the site of a primary tumor, and the primary draining lymph node or sentinel node is identified and removed for histopathological examination. Recent interest is being generated to examine the efficacy of sentinel node biopsy for intra-abdominal malignancy. Laparoscopy is well suited for the task because it could allow for both injection of the marker agent (dye or radioactive colloid) and biopsy of the lymph node. The radioimmunobiopsy is performed much like the sentinel node biopsy except that the radioactive molecule is linked to a monoclonal antibody directed against a tumor-specific antigen. The radioactive immunoglobins are injected intra-venously before surgery. At laparoscopy, specially designed detectors are inserted and „hot spots" of radioactivity identified. These areas are then biopsied and evaluated for metastases. Potentially, identification of nodal disease would improve staging and may alter treatment in a number of intra-abdominal diseases. The utility of this technique awaits further clinical trials.

Future Directions

Although still in its infancy, laparoscopic surgery continues to evolve at a rapid pace. Surgeons quickly mastered the set of basic skills needed to perform virtually every operation, but as the limits of minimal-access surgery are approached, its shortcomings stand out. As mentioned above, the current two-dimensional platform results in a severely reduced depth perception and lack of tactile sensation. Innovative concepts and tools are being developed to address these problems.

Two of the most exciting areas involve robotics and telesurgery. Robotics is the ability of an automatic apparatus to perform those functions normally performed by a human operator [17]. Teleoperation is the ability of a human operator to directly control an apparatus from some remote location. Telepresence is the ability of a human operator to receive information from an apparatus at a remote location in a fashion that allows the operator to perceive as though actually present at the procedure.

Robotic technology has already been used clinically in orthopedic practice. A robotic arm was used to assist hip replacement. In Europe, the first entirely robotically performed operation was a transurethral resection of the prostate, performed by Drs. Timoney and Wickam in 1991 [18]. Telepresent surgery extends this concept as well as attempting to achieve some tactile feedback. The setup consists of an operating table equipped with two CCD cameras that act sequentially to provide a feedback image that is „flicker-free". The remotely located surgeon sits at a workstation, wearing specially designed gloves, which provide sensory feedback from the robotic arm performing the surgery. The movements performed by the surgeon are matched by the robotic operator in real time, synchronized with the surgeon's movements made at the workstation. The ability to perceive weight, tension, and strength makes this technology an exciting and realistic possibility.

Virtual reality – a computer-driven, artificial, three-dimensional simulation of „real world" events – is also emerging as a new technology in laparoscopy, particularly in the training of inexperienced surgeons [19]. As laparoscopic surgery has integrated itself into the surgical arena over the past decade, the issue of training surgical residents or established surgeons with no laparoscopic experience has emerged as a problem. Virtual reality simulators can provide a safe and effective means for inexperienced surgeons to log numerous hours performing laparoscopic surgery. Although current technology does not yet provide a truly „real" experience, this will undoubtedly become an integral part in the teaching of laparoscopy.

References

1. Filipi CJ, Fitzgibbons RJ, Salerno GM (1991) In: Zucker KA (ed) Historical review: diagnostic laparoscopy to laparoscopic cholecystectomy and beyond, surgical laparoscopy. Quality Medical Publishing, Inc., St. Louis
2. Kelling G (1901) Über Oesophagoskopie, Gastroskopie und Colioskopie. Münch Med Wochenschr 49:21–24
3. Jacobaeus HC (1910) Über die Möglichkeit, die Zystoskopie bei Untersuchung seriöser Höhlungen anzuwenden. munch Med Wochenschr 57:2090–2092
4. Jacobaeus HC (1912) Über Laparo- und Thorakoskopie. Beitr Klin Tuberk 25:185–354
5. Bernheim BM (1911) Organoscopy: cystoscopy of the abdominal cavity. Ann Surg 53:764
6. Semm K (1987) Operative manual for endoscopic abdominal surgery (translated by ER Friederich). Year Book of Medical Publishers, Biermann Verlag, Köln
7. Eisenberg J (1966) Über eine Apparateur zur schonenden und kontrollierbaren Gasfüllung der Bauchhöhle für die Laparoskopie. Klin Wochenschr 44:593
8. Hasson HM (1978) Open laparoscopy vs. closed laparoscopy: a comparison of complication rates. Adv Planned Parenthood 13:41–50
9. Semm K (1984) Endoscopic intrabdominal surgery. Christian-Albrechts-Universität, Kiel, Germany
10. Dubois F, Berthelot G, Levard H (1989) Cholecystectomy par coelioscopy. Nouv Presse Med 18:980–982
11. Reddick EJ, Olsen D, Daniell J, Saye W, McKernan B, Miller W, Hoback M (1989) Laparoscopic laser cholecystectomy. Laser Med Surg News Adv Feb:38–40
12. Bismuth H, Castaing D, Garden OJ (1987) The use of operative ultrasound in surgery of primary liver tumors. World J Surg 11:610–614
13. Klotter HJ, Ruckert K, Kummerle F, Rothmund M (1987) The use of intraoperative sonography in endocrine tumors of the pancreas. World J Surg 11:635–641
14. Machi J, Sigel B (1996) Operative ultrasonography in general surgery. Am J Surg 172:15–20
15. Bakalakos EA, Burak WE Jr (1999) The radioimmunoguided surgery (RIGS) system as a diagnostic tool. Surg Oncol Clin N Am 8:129–144
16. Roselli M, Buonomo O, Piazza A, Guadagni F, Vecchione A, Brunetti E, Cipriani C, Amadei G, Nieroda C, Greiner JW, Casciani CU (1998) Novel clinical approaches in monoclonal antibody-based management in colorectal cancer patients: radioimmunoguided surgery and antigen augmentation. Semin Surg Oncol 15:254–262
17. Simon IB (1994) Future trends in minimal access surgery: telepresence surgery and virtual reality. In: Greene FL, Rosin RD (eds) Minimal access surgical oncology. Radcliffe Medical Press, Inc. New York, pp 183–186
18. Timoney A, Wickam JE (1991) The use of robots in surgery. The development of a frame for prostatectomy. J Endourol 5:165–168
19. Satava RM (1998) Transitioning to the future. J Am Coll Surg 186(6):691–692

Pathophysiological Aspects of the Pneumoperitoneum

P. HOHENBERGER

Historical Aspects

The first physician known to be interested in creating an abdominal wall filled with gas was Georg Kelling, a German surgeon. His interest was derived from the treatment of gastric hemorrhage, and his idea was to apply pressure on the bleeding organ by inducing a pneumoperitoneum. He first tested this procedure in dogs under general anesthesia and detected that intra-abdominal organs could be seen if he introduced a cystoscope for observation. His first publication on this idea was dated 1910.

In parallel to Kelling, Jacobaeus in Stockholm also used a pneumoperitoneum for diagnostic purposes in patients (see historical figures at the end of this chapter). Other early explorers of the abdominal cavity via a pneumoperitoneum were Berheim at Johns Hopkins Hospital in Baltimore and Ruddick and Zollikofer, with the latter applying CO_2 or room air.

Kalk, a German gastroenterologist, pioneered this procedure in the late 1920s. He developed new instruments and introduced a 30° oblique viewing endoscope in addition to the use of multiple trocars. He, and many hepatologists, used laparoscopy to explore the liver for a variety of diseases and to obtain biopsies under detailed view. The introduction of the so-called Veress needle was a milestone on the way to further distribution of this technique [1]. Laparoscopy became widely accepted in gynecology and hepatology and, particularly in Europe, was pushed forward by these disciplines. Berndt and Gütz were the first to use it in the pretherapeutic assessment of gastric cancer [2], and Semm and others started to switch over from gynecological operations to appendectomy and performed minor procedures in the field of general abdominal surgery [3–6]. The introduction of more elaborate and technically sophisticated camera models led the way to teaching of liver diseases by laparoscopic view. Perfect optical abdominal view facilitated repeated exploration of the liver during different stages of liver disease. The use of an intra-abdominal flashlight resulted in excellent photographs of abdominal organs and alterations to their surface [7]. This photographic technique resulted in extraordinarily precise and colorful illustrations better by far than any digitally equipped camera of today.

▌Complications During Laparoscopic Procedures

When a pneumoperitoneum was administered, often gas embolisms were suspected and/or observed. The main interest of surgeons when using pneumoperitoneal conditions was whether electrocoagulation could be used to control bleeding. To introduce noncombustible gas was of major interest. This question as well as the problem of gas embolisms, however, increased the interest in other pathophysiological conditions altered by administering the pneumoperitoneum (see also chapter on gasless laparoscopy). Beyond the different side effects of different types of gas (CO_2, helium, room air, NO_2) there are typical effects of high intra-abdominal pressure irrespective of the type of gas used. Generally, the heart rate increases and cardiac output drops. Furthermore, increased systemic vascular resistance and decreased splanchnic and renal blood flow can be detected. Depending on the abdominal pressure, changes in respiratory mechanisms are to be expected (see also page 5 'Gas pressure'). However, several authors have reported that a moderate increase in intra-abdominal pressure may lead to an increased effective cardiac filling pressure and increased cardiac output [8]. Clearly, high intra-abdominal pressure will decrease local tissue perfusion and regional blood flow of abdominal organs. All these changes are subject to preexisting cardiovascular dysfunction or pulmonary diseases.

Plasma catecholamine levels may be changed, and several groups reported that high intraperitoneal pressure resulted in significant metabolic acidosis as well as in increased levels of lactate [9]. The latter might be attributed to the impairment of regional tissue blood flow and/or oxygenation.

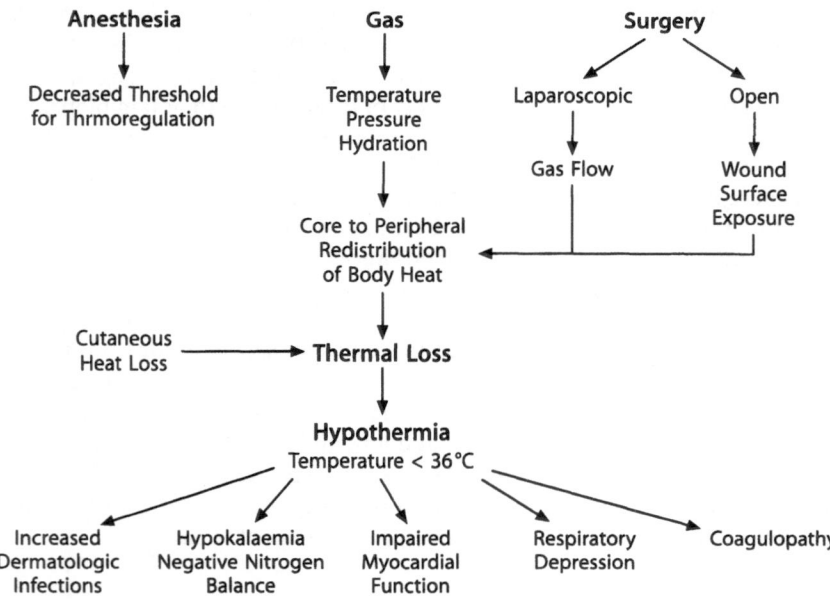

Fig. 1. Summary of the effects of gas temperature during laparoscopic procedures. (From [32])

Inert gases such as helium or argon may have advantages over CO_2 [10]. Solubility in water is decreased in comparison to CO_2, but the true role of these new gases is not yet fully explored because the cost-benefit ratio needs to be assessed and gas embolism under helium conditions might be much more deleterious than CO_2 emboli [11]. Some pathophysiological changes (pulmonary hypertension, increase of pulmonary vascular resistance) are less significantly observed under helium conditions than in the use of CO_2 [12]. The discussion of whether CO_2 is a vehicle for tumor cells and helium or argon are not is still in its initial stage.

Pneumoperitoneum with CO_2 results in disturbed temperature physiology with a significant fall in body core temperature over time (Fig. 1). As the majority of diagnostic laparoscopic procedures are finished within 1 h, no significant hypothermia should arise. The additional contribution of long-term laparoscopic surgical procedures under pneumoperitoneum condition might be counterbalanced by external body heating as it is generally performed in patients undergoing major operations with open laparotomy. Thus gas-warming insufflators have not proven to result in significant benefit to patients.

Changes in Hepatoportal Blood Flow

Except for liver cirrhosis associated with significant ascites, pneumoperitoneum is the most significant effector to hepatic and portal blood flow. Increased abdominal pressure induces an increased resistance to orthograde blood flow in the abdominal vessels. In this way, an increased pressure is also necessary to supply visceral organs with oxygenated blood. These data were mainly derived from critically ill patients [13]. As early as 1953, Olerud tried to calculate the resistance of a portal circulation under the circumstances of increased intra-abdominal pressure [14]. Subsequently, several studies in pigs and dogs proved that portal venous pressure is significantly increased as well as pressure in the inferior vena cava. Each of the investigators looked at different single organs to further study microcirculation. Taking these results together, blood flow in the inferior mesenteric artery, in the jejunal mucosa, as well as in the hepatic microcirculation is decreased (Fig. 2). There are significant correlations between the changes in intra-abdominal pressure and the concomitant changes (decrease) in hepatic artery blood flow, portal vein blood flow, and portal venous pressure. Under routine clinical circumstances, i.e., abdominal pressure of approximately 15 mmHg, the decrease of portal venous blood flow is approximately 25%–30% [15]. Portal venous pressure starts to increase if the abdominal pressures (IAP) exceeds 10 mmHg, whereas bile duct pressure continuously is correlated with intra-abdominal pressure. As a result, bile production is decreased.

The effects are probably due not only to increased mechanical pressure but also to hormonal influences including catecholamine and angiotensin. In women undergoing laparoscopic gynecological procedures, increased levels of vasopressin were found [16]. Additionally, the role of hypercapnia must be considered because an elevated pCO_2 yields a vasoconstrictive response in the mesenteric artery.

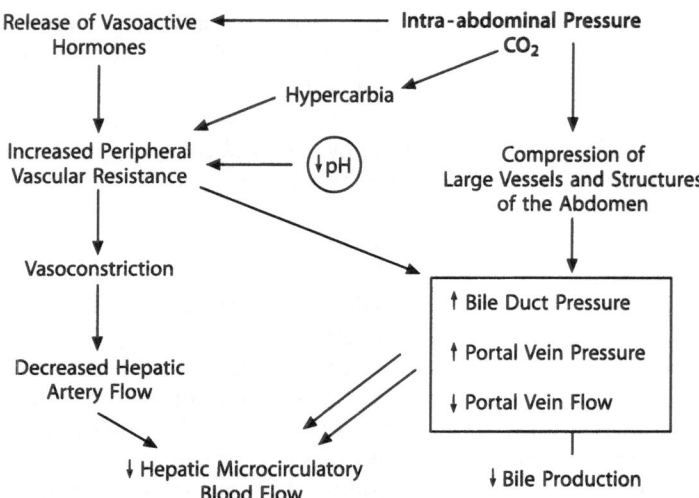

Fig. 2. Effects of elevated intra-abdominal pressure on the liver caused by direct mechanical pressure. (From [32])

Hepatorenal syndromes are rarely described under pneumoperitoneal circumstances [17], and it was suspected that compression of the liver and renal vasculature by elevated IAP was the cause.

Changes in Renal Blood Flow and Function

Acute renal failure in association with elevated IAP without severe disturbance of liver function has also been described. Normally, changes of renal function under the influence of pneumoperitoneum are less threatening. However, IAP is thought to induce an abdominal compartment syndrome [18] particularly concerning organs located in the retroperitoneum. The kidney and its vasculature might be severely affected already by intra-abdominal bleeding, ileus, hemorrhagic pancreatitis, or ascites.

During laparoscopic procedures with pneumoperitoneum renal blood flow might be disturbed easily. More than 80% of the renal blood flow perfuses the outer cortex of the kidney. Cardiac output as well as renal vascular resistance contribute to maintaining adequate renal blood flow. As is widely known, autoregulatory resistance is responsible to maintain an adequate intrarenal blood flow. The glomerular filtration process results in approximately 20% of the renal plasma flow being filtered.

There are very few clinical studies on renal hemodynamic effects of increased IAP. Data mainly derive from emergency patients and focus on the monitoring of urine output, assessing crush kidney syndrome and/or serum creatinine levels. Beyond affecting cardiac output, IAP might negatively influence renal blood flow because of compression of the renal cortex. Renal venous pressure might increase by obstructing the renal venous outflow in the retroperitoneum. Whether hormonal or neural influences are a general reaction to operative stress or selectively induced by the pneumoperitoneum remains a matter of discussion.

From animal experiments it could be shown that in contrast to the blood flow in the bowel there is no decrease of perfusion of the renal cortex if cardiac output is affected solely by increased IAP. This experience from canine models demonstrates that there might be a very different response of the visceral splanchnic vascular bed in comparison to the renal vasculature [19]. In a porcine model [20] clinical conditions were reproduced very accurately: CO_2 pneumoperitoneum was used at 15 mmHg, and renal cortex perfusion was assessed by laser-Doppler flowmetry. After 15 mmHg of abdominal pressure was applied, renal tissue perfusion was decreased to 40% of its initial values but returned immediately to the preinsufflation level if the pressure was released. Monitoring urine production might be inadequate to detect those changes because ureteral compression by increased IAP could be the responsible cause. Experimental data using an abdominal pressure of 80 mmHg reported an elevation of plasma ADH to more than twice the baseline levels. However, this degree of IAP is outside the clinical routine. More recent data show that at an IAP of 25 mmHg plasma renin activity as well as aldosterone were significantly increased in comparison to baseline values.

Given these findings, a close monitoring of renal function is mandatory, but there are no convincing data that pneumoperitoneum at 15 mmHg for approximately 2 h will lead to severe kidney damage.

Alterations of the Cardiopulmonary System

Experience had to be accumulated with alterations of the gas exchange and cardiac function when developments of laparoscopy resulted in timely extended operations. Initially, laparoscopy aimed at examining the lower pelvis during gynecological procedures and elevating the anterior abdominal wall to create a big cavity was not a significant part of the procedure [4-6]. The anti-Trendelenburg position removed the small bowel from the lower pelvis, giving view to the area of interest. However, during staging laparoscopy for gastrointestinal tract cancers or ovarian malignancies, rather high abdominal pressure is initiated and maintained for a considerable amount of time to provide better access to the retrogastric space and to thoroughly explore the surface of the diaphragm. Considering the small bowel and all subcavities of the abdomen, total peritoneal surface exceeds 2 m². From that point of view, it is not astonishing that significant resorption of CO_2 takes place via intercellular openings between mesothelial tissue of the parietal and visceral peritoneum. This might severely influence gas-exchange in the pulmonary system, particularly in patients suffering from chronic pulmonary diseases. It must be borne in mind that, for example, patients with esophageal cancer often have significant comorbidity in terms of chronic obstructive bronchitis or nicotine abuse. Elderly patients with pancreatic cancer might suffer from emphysema or have had pneumonia or tuberculosis earlier in life.

Absorption of gaseous molecules is predominantly by diffusion (Fig. 3) [21]. The peritoneal membrane, preperitoneal space, and capillary membrane enable

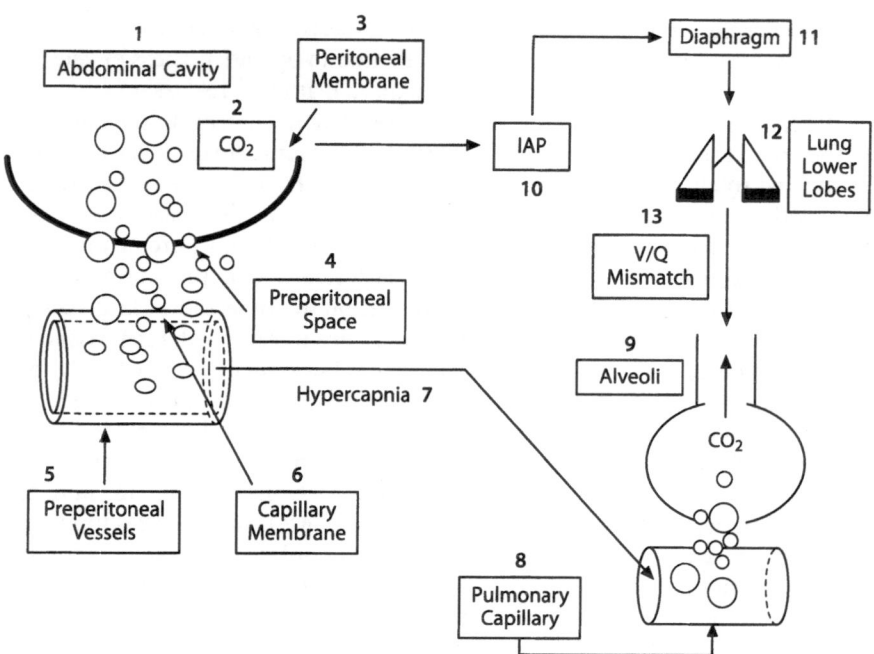

Fig. 3. The peritoneal cavity (*1*) is able to absorb gaseous molecules (*2*) by diffusion. Through the peritoneal membrane (*3*), preperitoneal space (*4*) and capillary membrane (*6*), carbon dioxide molecules can enter the peritoneal vessels (*5*), causing hypercapnia (*7*) by increasing the carbon dioxide blood tension. As a compensation, excretion of carbon dioxide through the alveoli will be increased (*8, 9*). When applying carbon dioxide pneumoperitoneum, intra-abdominal pressure (*IAP, 10*) will increase simultaneously, causing diminished excursion of the diaphragm (*11*) and compression of the lower lung lobes (*12*), resulting in decreased tidal volume and a ventilation-perfusion mismatch (*13*) with increased shunt and dead space volume. (From [32])

CO_2 molecules to enter peritoneal vessels, resulting in hypercapnia by increasing the carbon dioxide blood tension (pCO_2). Logically, excretion of CO_2 through the alveoli is increased. CO_2 pneumoperitoneum increases intra-abdominal pressure resulting in a diminished excursion of the diaphragm. Segmental atelectasis of the lower lung segments with decreased tidal volume, increased shunt, and dead space volume is the final result [22].

Hypercapnia is the key mechanism to both pulmonary and cardiovascular changes during laparoscopy. The high partial pressure difference between the intra-abdominal CO_2 pneumoperitoneum and pCO_2 in peritoneal vessels results in carrying CO_2 by circulation to the lung, where it is excreted. Plasma CO_2 concentration decreases, and the gas molecules are replaced by CO_2 emerging from red blood cells. Because CO_2 is capable of penetrating all cell membranes, it can exert systemic toxic effects of excretion and enzymatic transformation of the gas into the stomach or bone. Furthermore, activation of buffer systems in blood and kidney are accelerated. Insufflation of the pneumoperitoneal cavity results in disten-

Fig. 4. Algorithm for respiratory monitoring during laparoscopic procedures. *PEEP*, positive end-expiratory pressure; *Sat*, saturation. (From [32])

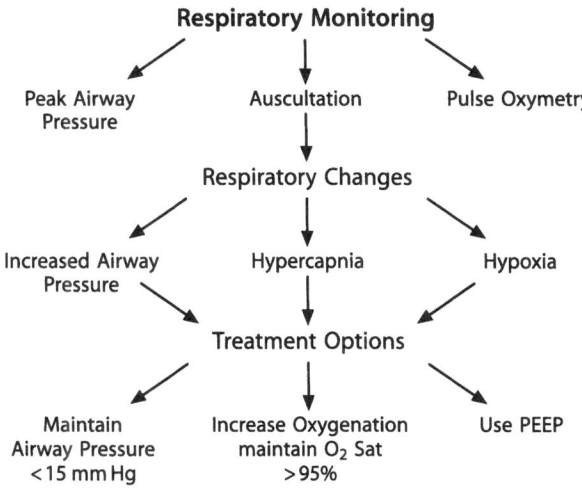

sion and significantly affects mechanically supported ventilation. The number of poorly ventilated alveoli increases, resulting in an increased ventilation-perfusion mismatch. Mild hypercapnia can cause sympathic stimulation that leads to an increase in heart rate and peripheral vasoconstriction. However, severe hypercapnia can exert a negative inotropic effect on the heart with decreased left ventricular function. As part of a randomized trial, ventilatory and arterial blood gas changes were assessed during open (n=30) and laparoscopic (n=30) cholecystectomy [23]. In comparison, no clinically significant changes in ventilation or blood gas values occurred during open cholecystectomy. However, laparoscopic cholecystectomy required a substantial but variable increase in minute ventilation to compensate for CO_2 absorption from the peritoneum (Fig. 4).

In patients with preexisting lung emphysema, expiration is already impaired by enlarged dead spaces. Hypoventilation is the result as airway ductuli are collapsing and dead space increases. On the other hand, patients with restrictive pulmonary diseases show alveoli with fibrotic membranes and an impaired gas exchange by decreased lung compliance with the consequence of an increased arteriovenous shunt volume. From a clinical point of view, those patients already have an impaired CO_2 excretion ability and pneumoperitoneum further will increase retaining CO_2. As a consequence of the increased arterial pCO_2 respiratory acidosis develops. Breathing frequency as well as tidal volume must be increased as an effect of hypercapnia. To overcome this mechanism, the application of positive end-expiratory pressure (PEEP) ventilation seems to be advantageous; however, CO_2 pneumoperitoneum in patients with preexisting lung disease should be limited to operation times as short as possible.

The hemodynamic changes associated with increased intra-abdominal pressure have already been stressed. Beyond the systemic effects of the insufflation gas, mechanical effects of increased intra-abdominal pressure must be taken into account. The negative inotropic effect of severe hypercapnia is the most prominent link that deserves attention. The hemodynamic change is most often ob-

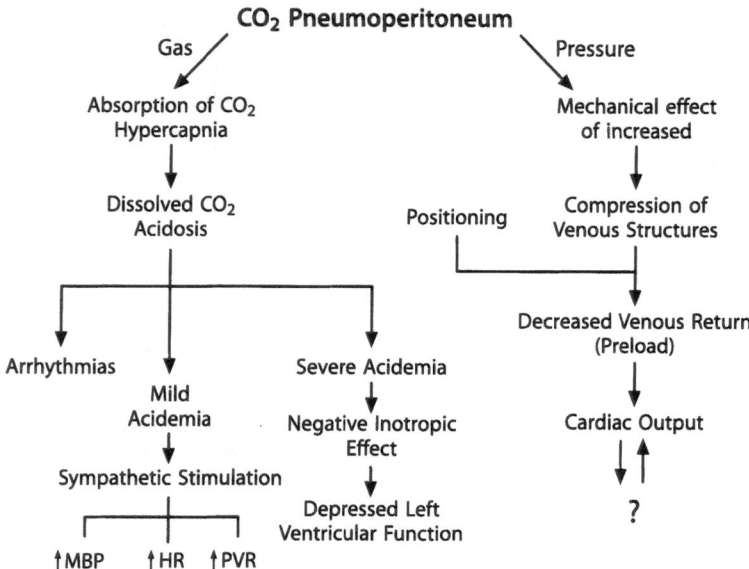

Fig. 5. Possible effects of gas and pressure of pneumoperitoneum. *MBP*, mean blood pressure; *HR*, heart rate; *PVR*, pulmonary venous pressure; *IAP*, intra-abdominal pressure. (From [32])

served as decrease in stroke volume with a compensatory tachycardia to maintain the cardiac index at baseline level. As in patients with preexisting lung disease, patients with limited cardiovascular compensatory mechanism also might be adversely affected by a timely extended pneumoperitoneum. During surgical procedures positioning of the patient is often changed from a Trendelenburg into an anti-Trendelenburg position and from a right-sided to a left-sided position, and often both extreme positionings (i.e., supine + right-sided) are combined. This might severely affect the intravascular volume status and, as a consequence, central filling pressures. All studies performed on humans [3, 24–26] show that cardiac output decreases and blood pressure increases as an effect of CO_2 pneumoperitoneum. It is worth mentioning that animal experiments yielded different results (Fig. 5).

Patients with high-risk cardiac disease (ASA category III or IV) may be at considerable risk of coronary ischemia. The problem of significant cardiovascular comorbidity is aggravated by the fact that volume loading to intraoperatively overcome decrease of venous return flow to the heart must be performed with caution. According to literature data [26] mixed venous oxygen saturation is the most sensitive parameter. Alternatively, insufflating gases are evaluated to avoid the physiological effects of CO_2, especially regarding acid-base and hormonal changes.

Mechanisms of gas embolism during laparoscopy are rather easy to understand. However, the true incidence of gas embolism is unknown. The incidence assessed during gynecological laparoscopies in the 1970s seemed to be rather high [27]. Also, in patients undergoing laparoscopic cholecystectomy, CO_2 embolism was observed in the majority of patients by transesophageal echocardiogram (TEE) [28]. However, all those events occurred without major changes in cardiorespiratory status. To result in a significant cardiorespiratory event, a large amount of CO_2 must enter the venous circulation with mechanical occlusion of the right heart or outflow tract of the right ventricle. Impaired venous return or cor pulmonale results in elevated central venous pressure, hypoxia, and left ventricular failure. Case reports on episodes of significant gas embolism report brachycardia, cyanosis, and rapid cardiovascular collapse as the leading symptoms. By TEE, CO_2 bubbles in the right atrium and ventricle can be detected, but because of the rather long intravascular route after being absorbed by peritoneal vessels the majority of CO_2 bubbles might be already dissolved when entering the right atrium. The most likely etiology of gas embolism therefore arises from venous injury during laparoscopic dissection. The danger is probably underestimated by surgeons unaware of the fact that even a minor venous leakage might be the source of major amounts of CO_2 absorption under 15-mmHg pneumoperitoneum.

Subcutaneous emphysema as well as pneumomediastinum are rather rare events; however, they depend on the operative manipulations performed [29–31] In case of tumors arising at the esophagogastric junction, exposure of the tumor area already might open up interstitial spaces to the posterior mediastinum. A tension pneumothorax is unlikely to develop because of the equilibration between pleural and peritoneal cavity and standardized and limited insufflation pressures. Furthermore, as long as the pleural cavity is not open, CO_2 gas bubbles may move their way through the posterior mediastinum, finally becoming noticeable or visible at the supraclavicular region.

Hemodynamic Changes to the Lower Limbs

Increased abdominal pressure might also influence blood flow in iliac, femoral, and popliteal veins. Using Doppler ultrasound for measurements at the extremity level and transesophageal Doppler to assess central flow it could be demonstrated that after induction of a pneumoperitoneum blood flow in the common femoral vein decreases significantly [32]. Laparoscopic cholecystectomy as well as fundoplicatio are the most common procedures during which these investigations have been performed. Peak systolic velocity of femoral venous blood flow drops from a mean of 6 cm/s to 4.2 cm/s and end diastolic velocity from 3.5 cm/s to 2.7 cm/s [33]. After control of changes in cardiac output, stroke volume, blood pressure, and pulse rate it was argued that the decreased venous flow places the patients at increased risk for deep vein thrombosis. Lymphatic compression devices have been used to compensate the adverse effects of pneumoperitoneum and intraoperatively, a repetitive, pneumatic compression of the muscles of the lower limb is administered [33–35]. This approach seems logical; however, at present only scarce data are available. Recommendations to use such a device for patients at risk for perioperative complications must be taken with caution because it is not clear that artificial and sequential pulsatile venous blood flow would not adversely affect those patients with preexisting cardiopulmonary risk factors. Furthermore, the risk of deep vein thrombosis can hardly be estimated. The incidence of pulmonary embolism and deep vein thrombosis during laparoscopic cholecystectomy were reported at 0.64% [36]. Whether these results can be adapted to patients suffering from cancer – incidence for staging laparoscopy – remains unclear. All patients require low-molecular-weight heparin in addition to any mechanical devices.

In conclusion, laparoscopy using standard CO_2 pneumoperitoneum and an intra-abdominal pressure limit of 15 mmHg regularly induces significant alterations to the cardiopulmonary system, hepatoportal blood flow, and renal and mesenteric perfusion. If the procedure is intended just for staging purposes dramatic side effects beyond pathophysiological adaptations must not be expected. Thorough preoperative work-up of the patients by an experienced anesthesiologist and by subspecialists of internal medicine should be performed in those patients with known comorbidity to their malignant disease. Proceeding from staging laparoscopy to definitive, minimally invasive surgical procedures requires further detailed diagnostic measures to ensure minimal risk for the patient.

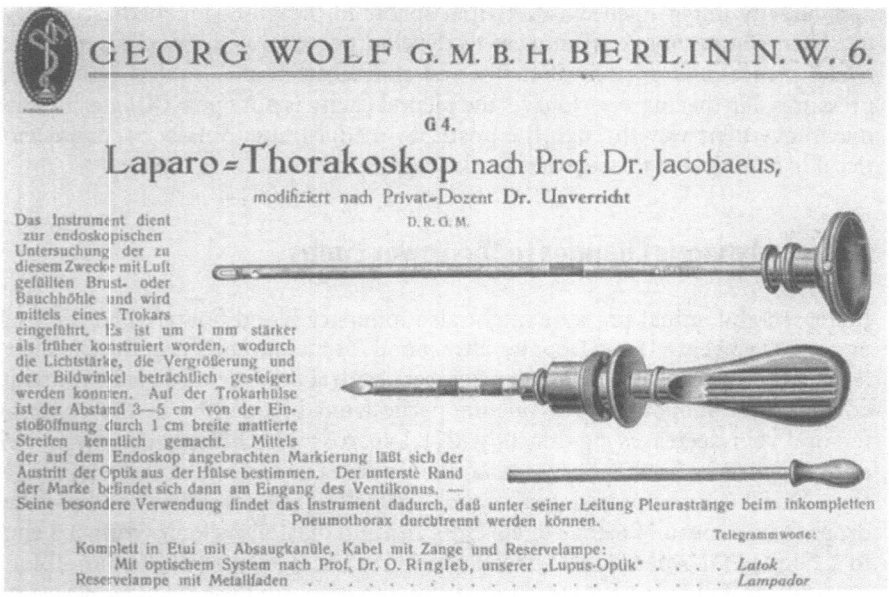

Advertisement for the „laparo-/thoracoscope" manufactured by Wolf in Germany in 1927. In comparison to the original developed by Jacobaeus in 1910 this new laparoscope had been changed from 4 mm to 5 mm diameter by this way improving view and illumination

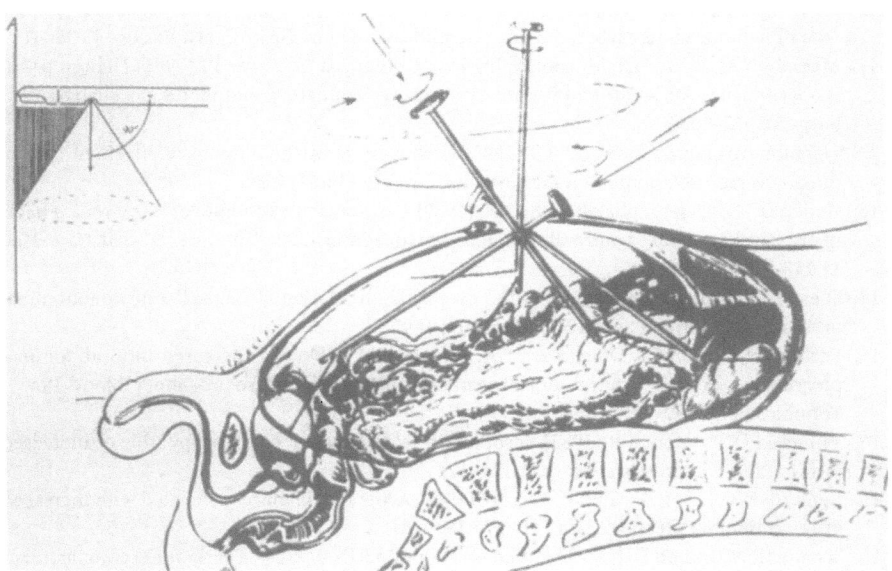

Original drawing to illustrate the exploration of different intraabdominal quadrants via a 90°
side-view optic by Jacobaeus in 1913 (taken from: „Über Laparo- und Thorakoskopie, Dr. H. C.
Jacobaeus, Sonerdruck aus der Reihe „Beiträge zur Klinik der Tuberkulose, XXXV.Bd, Heft 2,
Verlag Curt Kabitzsch, Würzburg, 1913)

▌ References

1. Veress J (1938) Neues Instrument zur Ausführung von Brust- oder Bauchpunktionen und
   Pneumothoraxbehandlung. Dtsch Med Wochenschr 64:1480–1482
2. Berndt H, Gütz HJ (1965) Laparoskopie bei Magenkrebs. Z Gastroenterol 3:317–320
3. Motew M, Ivankovich AD, Bieniarz J, Albrecht RF, Zahed B, Scommegna A (1973)
   Cardiovascular effects and acid-base and blood gas changes during laparoscopy. Am J
   Obstet Gynecol 115:1002–1012
4. Lewis DG, Ryder W, Burn N, Wheldon JT, Tacchi D (1972) Laparoscopy – an investigation
   during spontaneous ventilation with halothane. Br J Anaesth 44:685–691
5. Semm K (1988) Die pelviskopische Appendektomie. [Pelviscopic appendectomy]. Dtsch
   Med Wochenschr 113:3–5
6. Semm K (1988) Sichtkontrollierte Peritoneumperforation zur operativen Pelviskopie.
   [Visible control of peritoneal perforation in surgical pelviscopy]. Geburtshilfe Frauenheilkd
   48:436–439
7. Henning H, Lightdale CJ, Look D (1994) Color atlas of diagnostic laparoscopy. Thieme,
   Stuttgart New York
8. Liu SY, Leighton T, Davis I, Klein S, Lippmann M, Bongard F (1991) Prospective analysis of cardiopulmonary responses to laparoscopic cholecystectomy. J Laparoendosc Surg 1:241–246
9. Taura P, Lopez A, Lacy AM, Anglada T, Beltran J, Fernandez-Cruz L et al. (1998) Prolonged
   pneumoperitoneum at 15 mmHg causes lactic acidosis. Surg Endosc 12:198–201

10. Neuberger TJ, Andrus CH, Wittgen CM, Wade TP, Kaminski DL (1996) Prospective comparison of helium versus carbon dioxide pneumoperitoneum. Gastrointest Endosc 43:38–41
11. McMahon AJ, Baxter JN, Murray W, Imrie CW, Kenny G, O'Dwyer PJ (1994) Helium pneumoperitoneum for laparoscopic cholecystectomy: ventilatory and blood gas changes. Br J Surg 81:1033–1036
12. Leighton TA, Liu SY, Bongard FS (1993) Comparative cardiopulmonary effects of carbon dioxide versus helium pneumoperitoneum. Surgery 113:527–531
13. Cullen DJ, Coyle JP, Teplick R, Long MC (1989) Cardiovascular, pulmonary, and renal effects of massively increased intra-abdominal pressure in critically ill patients. Crit Care Med 17:118–121
14. Olerud S (1953) Experimental studies on portal circulation at increased intra-abdominal pressure. Acta Physiol Scand 30 [Suppl 109]:1–95
15. Diebel LN, Wilson RF, Dulchavsky SA, Saxe J (1992) Effect of increased intra-abdominal pressure on hepatic arterial, portal venous, and hepatic microcirculatory blood flow. J Trauma 33:279–282
16. Viinamki O, Punnonen R (1982) Vasopressin release during laparoscopy: role of increased intra-abdominal pressure. Lancet 1:175–176
17. Richards WO, Scovill W, Shin B, Reed W (1983) Acute renal failure associated with increased intra-abdominal pressure. Ann Surg 197:183–187
18. Schein M, Wittmann DH, Aprahamian CC, Condon RE (1995) The abdominal compartment syndrome: the physiological and clinical consequences of elevated intra-abdominal pressure. J Am Coll Surg 180:745–753
19. Harman PK, Kron IL, McLachlan HD, Freedlender AE, Nolan SP (1982) Elevated intra-abdominal pressure and renal function. Ann Surg 196:594–597
20. Chiu AW, Chang LS, Birkett DH, Babayan RK (1996) A porcine model for renal hemodynamic study during laparoscopy. J Surg Res 60:61–68
21. Tsilibary EC, Wissig SL (1983) Lymphatic absorption from the peritoneal cavity: regulation of patency of mesothelial stomata. Microvasc Res 25:22–39
22. Wittgen CM, Andrus CH, Fitzgerald SD, Baudendistel LJ, Dahms TE, Kaminski DL (1991) Analysis of the hemodynamic and ventilatory effects of laparoscopic cholecystectomy. Arch Surg 126:997–1000
23. McMahon AJ, Baxter JN, Kenny G, O'Dwyer PJ (1993) Ventilatory and blood gas changes during laparoscopic and open cholecystectomy. Br J Surg 80:1252–1254
24. McLaughlin JG, Scheeres DE, Dean RJ, Bonnell BW (1995) The adverse hemodynamic effects of laparoscopic cholecystectomy. Surg Endosc 9:121–124
25. Marshall RL, Jebson PJ, Davie IT, Scott DB (1972) Circulatory effects of peritoneal insufflation with nitrous oxide. Br J Anaesth 44:1183–1187
26. Safran D, Sgambati S, Orlando R (1993) Laparoscopy in high-risk cardiac patients. Surg Gynecol Obstet 176:548–554
27. Phillips J, Keith D, Hulka J, Hulka B, Keith L (1976) Gynecologic laparoscopy in 1975. J Reprod Med 16:105–117
28. Cottin V, Delafosse B, Viale JP (1996) Gas embolism during laparoscopy: a report of seven cases in patients with previous abdominal surgical history. Surg Endosc 10:166–169
29. Loffer FD, Pent D (1975) Indications, contraindications and complications of laparoscopy. Obstet Gynecol Surv 30:407–427
30. Prystowsky JB, Jericho BG, Epstein HM (1993) Spontaneous bilateral pneumothorax-complication of laparoscopic cholecystectomy. Surgery 114:988–992
31. Marcus DR, Lau WM, Swanstrom LL (1996) Carbon dioxide pneumothorax in laparoscopic surgery. Am J Surg 171:464–466

32. Reymond MA, Christen Y, Morel P, Köckerling F (1998) Pneumoperitoneum-related circulatory changes of the lower extremities. In: Rosenthal RJ, Friedman RL, Phillips EH (eds) The pathophysiology of pneumoperitoneum. Springer, New York, pp 28–41
33. Alishahi S, Francis N, Crofts S, Duncan L, Bickel A, Cuschieri A (2001) Central and peripheral adverse hemodynamic changes during laparoscopic surgery and their reversal with a novel intermittent sequential pneumatic compression device. Ann Surg 233:176–182
34. Jorgensen JO, Lalak NJ, North L, Hanel K, Hunt DR, Morris DL (1994) Venous stasis during laparoscopic cholecystectomy. Surg Laparosc Endosc 4:128–133
35. Jorgensen JO, Gillies RB, Lalak NJ, Hunt DR (1994) Lower limb venous hemodynamics during laparoscopy: an animal study. Surg Laparosc Endosc 4:32–35
36. Jorgensen JO, Hanel K, Lalak NJ, Hunt DR, North L, Morris DL (1993) Thromboembolic complications of laparoscopic cholecystectomy. BMJ 306:518–519

Risk of Port Site Metastases

V. Paolucci · R. Linker · C.N. Gutt

Laparoscopy has become more and more popular in the treatment and staging of intra-abdominal tumors, especially in gastroenterology but also in gynecology and general surgery. Oncological patients should also benefit from a minimally invasive approach. However, at the beginning of the establishment of this process in the field of cancer surgery, laparoscopy was overshadowed by specific problems such as tumor recurrence at the site of insertion of the laparoscope (port site metastases) and rapid intraperitoneal tumor dissemination [1–3]. Therefore, the fact of postlaparoscopic metastatic disease at trocar sites and possible enlarged intra-abdominal tumor dissemination slowed down widespread employment of laparoscopic techniques to resect malignant tumors. Many reports have been published since this complication first occurred. Most of these reports show the recurrence of port site metastases after laparoscopic resection of colorectal cancer, diagnostic laparoscopy for digestive cancer, or removal of gallbladder with occult cancer [2]. Incidences of port site metastases associated with laparoscopic colorectal surgery as high as 21% were quoted [2]. These results may be due to poor surgical techniques during early experience in the field. In contrast, some recent studies of larger patient pools have documented incidences of port site recurrences as low as 2% [4–6]. Looking at conventional open surgery in colorectal malignancy we see a very rare incidence of abdominal recurrence. Here incidence is quoted as 0.69% or higher, with 3.3% in patients that were operated conventionally by laparotomy and in whom recurrences were recorded 3 months after operation [7, 8]. By the end of 1997 there were 164 published cases of laparoscopic and thoracoscopic tumor seeding.

Literature Review

To review all reported cases of port site recurrence, a search of the medical literature through December 1997 was performed. To date, 164 cases of port site recurrences after endoscopic procedures in patients with known or even unsuspected cancers have been reported in 90 publications. Table 1 gives a summary of all cases divided into the different types of surgery. The majority of the reported implantation metastases were related to laparoscopy for digestive tumors (108/164). Of these, 96 appeared after therapeutic laparoscopy and 12 after diagnostic procedures.

Table 1. Neoplastic port site recurrence after laparoscopic procedures (n=164)

Type of laparoscopy	Therapeutic	Diagnostic	Total
Gynecology	1	28	29
Abdominal	96	12	108
Cholecystectomy	46		
Colorectal	47		
Gastric procedures	1	5	
Others	2	7	
Thoracic			23
Urology	2	2	4

Forty-eight percent (46/96) of port site metastases occurred after laparoscopic cholecystectomy for unsuspected gallbladder carcinoma. In all cases the primary diagnosis was cholelithiasis or cholecystitis. Even during operation there was no visual evidence of abnormalities, and histological examination of the specimens first revealed the carcinoma. In most cases the carcinoma infiltrated the whole gallbladder wall involving the serosal surface, and in some cases, even the adjacent tissue was invaded (stage III and IV, respectively). However, seven patients had a primary T2 carcinoma of the gallbladder, and one female patient developed port site metastases 23 months after laparoscopic cholecystectomy for a T1G1 gallbladder carcinoma. Nearly all patients (except 6) were older than 50 years. Of the 46 patients who developed port site metastases, 24 died within 2–19 months and 6 were still alive 4–30 months after cholecystectomy. The follow-up of the remaining 16 patients is unknown. In two cases, laparoscopic cholecystectomy was performed for gallbladder disease and later adenocarcinoma of the colon was discovered. The patients underwent an open right hemicolectomy and developed port site recurrences of the colon carcinoma 8 and 9 months later, respectively. A 71-year-old male patient developed a port site metastasis of an adenocarcinoma 6 months after laparoscopic cholecystectomy, although histological examination of the gallbladder did not find any malignancy. Autopsy showed an adenocarcinoma of the pancreas. Forty-nine percent (47/96) of the port site metastases appeared after laparoscopy for Duke's A (n=3), B (n=11), C (n=24), and D (n=1) colorectal cancer. In eight patients the tumor stage was described. The follow-up of most patients was unknown. Three other cases of port site recurrences have been described after laparoscopy for gastric, pancreatic, and esophageal carcinoma.

In the patients who developed port site recurrences after diagnostic laparoscopy for malignancy, the procedure was performed either to take biopsies or for staging of pancreatic or gastric carcinoma. Of 12 patients, follow-up is unknown in 1 case, 1 patient was still alive after 67 months, and the remaining 10 patients died within 1–10 months.

International Survey

A survey with members of the German Society of Surgery, the Swiss Society of Endoscopic Surgeons, and the Austrian Society of Endoscopic Surgeons was carried out to assess the dimension of the problem of port site metastases.

A first mailing, which included a cover letter that explained the purpose of the study and a one-page survey, was mailed in the winter of 1995–1996 to the 1,052 surgical department chairmen members of the three societies. The members were asked whether or not they had observed cases of port site metastasis after laparoscopy in patients with unsuspected or known malignancy. The questionnaire was structured in such a way as not to be too detailed or complicated, to ensure a sufficient number of responses.

Because of the unexpectedly high number of positive reports, and the marked interest in the „tumor seeding" problem demonstrated by the participants, in spring 1996 a second mailing was sent to all of the 448 responders. The second, quite detailed, questionnaire was structured to focus on the laparoscopic practice of every institution, incidence of tumor dissemination, localization, time interval between laparoscopic procedure and metastatic event, and stage of the primary tumor. The specific questions we asked were: (1) whether the specimen was damaged during surgery, (2) whether a protection bag was used during extraction, (3) demographic data, (4) further therapy, and (5) long-term outcome after laparoscopic surgery. Each case of documented recurrence was recorded separately with regard to demographic data, tumor stage at laparoscopy, time and site of metastasis, follow-up, and outcome.

Usable data were returned from 443 hospitals in Germany (n=401), Switzerland (n=18), Austria (n=17), Hungary (n=4), and Turkey (n=3). Three hundred fifty respondents (80%) neither saw any suspicious tumor seeding after laparoscopy nor referred to anecdotal cases. Four participants presented insufficiently documented cases (n=4), which could not be used. Eighty-nine respondents (20%) had observed cases of tumor spreading, consisting of abdominal wall metastases or surprisingly rapid signs of peritoneal carcinomatosis after laparoscopic procedures with CO_2 pneumoperitoneum, and documented them sufficiently. The number of metastatic cases identified at individual hospitals ranged from 1 to 4 with a total of 109 patients. Table 2 lists the general data of our survey.

Table 2. International survey. Laparoscopic tumor dissemination occurrence at 443 hospitals

Gallbladder cancer	Patients
Port site metastases	70
Peritoneal carcinomatosis	6
Colorectal cancer	
Port site metastases	16
Peritoneal carcinomatosis	3
Metastases of other types of cancer	14
Total	109

Metastases of Nonapparent Gallbladder Cancer

A total of 117,840 laparoscopic cholecystectomies for stone disease were reported. Unsuspected gallbladder cancer was diagnosed in 409 cases, by microscopic examination of the specimen or on the basis of later appearance of gallbladder cancer metastases. The incidence of nonapparent gallbladder carcinoma in our survey was 0.35%. After laparoscopic cholecystectomy for nonapparent carcinoma of the gallbladder, 70 patients (17.1%) were recognized to have at least one port site metastasis. A total of 86 differently located port site metastases were observed in 70 patients during the postoperative course after laparoscopic cholecystectomy. In seven patients, tumor recurrence was found simultaneously in more than one port site, and in eight cases peritoneal carcinosis was also present at the time of the first recurrence. The port used for gallbladder extraction was the most common site of recurrence (n=49); 37 recurrences, however, appeared in a port site that had not been used for specimen retrieval. In at least 8 cases (11.5%) a protective plastic bag was used for extraction of the gallbladder, and in 59 patients (84.3%) the gallbladder was not opened during the laparoscopic procedure or extraction. In nine patients with a nonapparent T1 tumor of the gallbladder, the specimen was removed intact. In three patients with a T2 tumor, the gallbladder was removed both intact and with the assistance of a protective bag.

The time of the first clinical tumor recurrence after laparoscopic cholecystectomy was a median of 180 days with a range from 14 to 880 days. At the time of cholecystectomy 13 patients showed a T1 tumor, all but 3 with cancer invasion beyond the muscularis mucosae. Thirty-six patients (51%) had a T2 gall bladder cancer, in four cases with lymph node metastases. There were three cases of direct tumor invasion of the liver (T3) and only one patient with a T4 tumor. In 13 cases, primary microscopic examination detected no signs of malignancy and gallbladder cancer was diagnosed later based on histological examination of port site metastases (n=4) and on reexamination of the gallbladder after detection of the metastases (n=9). In most cases, the N category (lymph node involvement) could not be assessed because a second operation with lymphadenectomy was not performed. Fifty-five patients had already died at the time data sampling was stopped. The survival time after laparoscopy was a median of 360 days (range 98–1,100 days). Fifteen patients were still alive 90–1,400 days after cholecystectomy. The overall 2-year survival was 18.5%.

In six patients (1.5%) early peritoneal carcinomatosis was the first recurrence, 22–270 days (median 120 days) after laparoscopic cholecystectomy in the presence of unsuspected gallbladder carcinoma. In two cases, peritoneal carcinosis was found at the moment of planned reoperation after histological detection of carcinoma of the gallbladder, 22 and 23 days, respectively, after laparoscopy. In one patient with a differentiated pT1 carcinoma, diffuse peritoneal involvement occurred 4 months after laparoscopy, and he died of tumor progression 1 month later. The survival of this small group was 240 days in median.

Metastases of Colorectal Cancer

A total of 412 laparoscopies in the presence of colon or rectal cancer have been reported. In 19 patients (4.6%) tumor seeding was observed. Sixteen (3.9%) of these patients had one or more port site and scar recurrences 90–750 days after laparoscopy with a median of 190 days. Ten patients had had a laparoscopic colon resection with curative intention. In three cases, palliative laparoscopic surgery was attempted because of liver and lung metastases. In one female patient, laparoscopic detachment of adhesions was performed 16 months after open right hemicolectomy for a pT3pN1M0 adenocarcinoma of the caecum. She developed a port site metastasis in the left subcostal region 90 days later and diffuse peritoneal carcinosis 3 months later. In three cases, the colon tumor did not have lymph node metastases at the time of laparoscopy. In two female patients right hemicolectomy was performed after laparoscopic inspection of the abdominal cavity. They had developed port site metastases in the lower right abdominal quadrant 7 and 23 months later, respectively. The site of recurrence was the minilaparotomy scar used for specimen extraction in 3 patients, the perineal scar in 1 patient, and one or two of the port sites, in 12 patients. The tumor specimen was intact and a protective plastic bag was used for tumor extraction in seven cases, in four cases no specimen was retrieved laparoscopically, in four cases the intact specimen was extracted without any wound protection, and in one case the opened tumor was retrieved without a plastic bag. Seven patients were already dead at the end of the inquiry, 190–630 days after laparoscopy (median of 360 days). Eight patients were alive 138 days to 3 years (median of 2 years) after laparoscopy, and there was one dropout.

Of the remaining three patients with unusual recurrence patterns but without port site metastases, one female patient developed diffuse peritoneal carcinosis, diagnosed 390 days after a laparoscopic sigmoid colon resection. In two cases, an extended carcinoma of the rectum and of the transverse colon, respectively, with diffuse peritoneal carcinosis was diagnosed, 80 and 270 days, respectively, after an uneventful laparoscopic cholecystectomy.

Metastases of Other Carcinomas

Port site metastases have been reported after diagnostic laparoscopy, with or without biopsy, for different abdominal carcinomas in seven cases (once followed by radical surgery), after laparoscopic gastroenterostomy for metastatic pancreatic cancer in two cases, and after laparoscopic cholecystectomy in the presence of nonapparent intra-abdominal malignancies in five cases. In three patients, two differently located port site recurrences were diagnosed simultaneously. The metastatic process appeared between 6 days and 3 years after laparoscopy (median of 70 days). Seven patients had tumor biopsies or diagnostic aspiration of intra-abdominal fluid through a separate cannula; in all but two of these patients, this was the site of recurrence. Seven patients were already dead by the time this survey was closed, 95 days to 3 years (with median of 225 days) after laparoscopy. Seven patients were still alive 90 days to 3 years (median of 185 days) after laparoscopy.

▌ Discussion

Laparoscopically assisted surgery for gastrointestinal and gynecologic cancer has been suggested to result in an earlier return of bowel function, earlier discharge of the patient from the hospital, and a more rapid return to work and activities of daily living [3, 9, 10]. However, the principal concern in treating patients for cancer is not short-term pain relief or the length of the scar but rather the optimal outcome for the patient. Although sufficient lymphadenectomy and adequate margins of resection have been achieved in series with selected patients [10–12], major concern exists about laparoscopic cancer treatment with regard to the long-term outcome [3, 13, 14]. In the setting of expanding oncological laparoscopy, the increasing number of case reports that have suggested the possibility of port site recurrence as well as peritoneal carcinomatosis after laparoscopy for malignant conditions still remains an obstacle [1–3, 15–18].

At the end of 1997, 164 cases of port site recurrence after laparoscopy or thoracoscopy had been reported. Most metastases occurred in patients with advanced disease, but an increasing number were found after operations for T1 and T2 gallbladder cancers as well as Duke's A and B colorectal cancers. In this clinical situation numerous editorials and reviews have concluded that laparoscopic surgery for cancer should not be performed outside controlled studies until there are enough data about the clinical importance of this complication.

Wound implantation is not a very new phenomenon. In 1983, Hughes et al. reported on wound recurrences after surgery. Laparotomy scar recurrence was seen after 13 of 1,600 operations, mainly accompanied with carcinomatosis. Isolated wound recurrence was seen in only 0.2% of patients. More recently, Reilly et al. reported on scar metastases after open surgery for colorectal cancer. In 26 (1.5%) of 1,711 patients wound recurrence was noted, but only 3 of the 1,711 patients (0.2%) were found to have an isolated scar recurrence without other metastatic locations. In contrast, an analysis of the laparoscopic colon cancer registry of the American Society of Colon and Rectal Surgeons has shown 5 cases of port site recurrence in a series of 480 cases (1.1%) followed for at least 12 months [19]. In a multicenter analysis including 1,333 diagnostic and therapeutic laparoscopies for cancer, Anderson et al. [20] showed a 6.7% rate of port site metastases after gallbladder and bile duct surgery and a 1.8% rate after colonic surgery. Even diagnostic laparoscopy has been associated with port site metastases in literature. Dehn and Cook [21] found an 11% port site recurrence rate in a series of 46 patients who underwent laparoscopy for different malignancies. However, the exact incidence of wound metastasis after laparoscopic surgery cannot be evaluated until the denominator of that number of procedures is known.

The survey of 443 hospitals addresses the incidence of this complication, based on 409 cases of nonapparent gallbladder cancer and 412 cases of colorectal cancer. Furthermore, 14 reports of port site metastases from other malignancies were collected. The response rate of 42% is similar to that of previous inquiries about complications of laparoscopic surgery [3, 14]. The results, however, do not represent the total incidence of laparoscopic tumor seeding, because not all clinics using laparoscopic techniques responded to the questionnaire. These numbers could be just the tip of the iceberg. According to the data, overall incidence of port site metastases after laparoscopic cholecystectomy for gall bladder cancer is 17.1% after a median time of 6 months. It is difficult to interpret the six cases (1.5%) of early peritoneal carcinomatosis without port site recurrence as a consequence of laparoscopy with any degree of certainty because intraperitoneal recurrence is a typical feature of gallbladder cancer [22, 23]. However, one feature of particular interest is that peritoneal tumor seeding presented in a median of 4 months, in two cases only 3 weeks, after cholecystectomy and, furthermore, in a patient with a differentiated T1 carcinoma.

The outcome for patients with port site metastases of a gallbladder carcinoma in this inquiry is poor. The overall 2-year survival rate of 18.5% is very low if we consider that all patients have had nonapparent and, at least 13 of them, a T1 carcinoma. In a series of 32 gallbladder carcinomas first diagnosed at microscopic examination after open cholecystectomy, Bergdahl [24] found a 22% 5-year and a 16% 10-year survival rate without any therapy other than cholecystectomy. In a more recent Japanese study on 98 patients with nonapparent carcinoma of the gallbladder operated on with conventional cholecystectomy, Shirai [25] found up to 90% 5-year survival for T2 and 100% 5-year survival for T1 tumors.

The potentially aggressive nature of such recurrences is evident. In the survey some port site recurrences and peritoneal carcinomatosis occurred within days or weeks after laparoscopic surgery. Other authors observed cases of very early recurrence, partly associated with a rapid deterioration in the course of the disease [1–4, 26–28]. In contrast, it is the current perception that wound recurrence after open cholecystectomy for primary nonapparent carcinoma of the gallbladder must be an exceptional event. During the literature search we did not find any of these complications between 1960 and 1996. The two reports mentioned discuss, respectively, 32 and 98 cases of gallbladder carcinoma, unrecognized before and at the time of operation and followed up for 10 and 8 years, respectively; neither described scar recurrence [24, 25]. Abdominal scar metastases of gallbladder cancer seem to be a specific complication of laparoscopy.

In contrast to convictions previously held [29] that the phenomenon of laparoscopic tumor seeding is essentially mechanical in origin and mainly depends on intraoperative accidents such as disruption of the gallbladder wall and spreading of tumor cells through the extraction or working port sites, our data show that the presence of mucosal tumor, intact specimen, and protective retrieval bag cannot exclude the port site metastasis. We must examine other more likely biologic causes, for instance, the physical influence of intra-abdominal pressure on tumor cell diffusion into tissue and direct chemical effects of CO_2 pneumoperitoneum on tumor cell growth or on local defense against tumor cell implantation.

Regarding tumor seeding after laparoscopy for colorectal cancer, the results of our inquiry confirm preexisting data from the literature. The 412 laparoscopies considered in patients with colorectal cancer showed an overall incidence of tumor seeding of 4.6%, with an incidence of port site metastases of 3.9%. Few authors have previously provided incidence figures. Fingerhut [16] reported the French experience of 92 laparoscopic resections for colon carcinoma and found the overall incidence of port site recurrence to be 3.2%. Prasad et al. [30] reported a 4% incidence of port site recurrence in a series of 50 patients. Berends et al. [31] noted three port metastases in 14 patients (21%). In 208 patients registered with laparoscopic colectomy, Ramos et al. [32] found three wound recurrences, two of them with peritoneal carcinomatosis (1.4%). Other authors with relatively small sample series [11] also could not observe any cases of unusual recurrence. Wexner [2] estimated the incidence of this complication, on the basis of published data, to be 4%. In our opinion, 4% could now be generally accepted as the overall rate for this complication. However, it is noteworthy that in our inquiry no patients with metastases or early peritoneal carcinomatosis had a T1 or T2 tumor, indicating that the incidence of laparoscopic tumor seeding could be much lower for early cancer and higher for advanced cancer. Nineteen cases of our series were quite advanced, and only four did not have metastatic lymph node involvement at the time of laparoscopy. The overall incidence of colorectal tumor seeding after laparoscopy seems to be three to four times higher than in open surgery. An analysis of the recurrence within laparotomy incisions after colonic tumor surgery was made in 1983 [7]. In their review of 1,603 resected patients, Hughes and colleagues identified 13 (0.8%) recurrences in operative sites; 8 of these occurred in Duke's B and 3 in Duke's C primary lesions. The most recent data on the frequency of wound recurrence in a population of high-risk patients, treated for cure and followed clinically on prospective randomized adjuvant therapy trials, were provided by Reilly and colleagues in 1996: 11 of 1,711 patients (0.6%) had documented incisional recurrences, 2 of them had primary stage Duke's B2, and 9 had primary stage Duke's C disease. The incidence of laparoscopic tumor seeding in our survey is higher than the published incidence of wound recurrence after laparotomy for colorectal cancer. This phenomenon, however, seems to be limited to tumors that have infiltrated the serosal layer. Furthermore, most recurrences occurred in patients with lymph node-positive disease.

Trocar port metastases have been described in the literature after laparoscopic biopsy for hepatocellular carcinoma [33], diagnostic laparoscopy in a patient with ascites and gastric cancer [34], laparoscopic cholecystectomy for an undiagnosed pancreatic carcinoma [35], and laparoscopic resection of unsuspected or low-malignant ovarian cancer [3, 17]. From at least one report, it is clear that direct tumor handling is not a prerequisite for trocar site implantation of metastases [35]. Even diagnostic procedures without tumor biopsy have been followed by tumor seeding [21, 35, 36]. Laparoscopic devices such as specimen bags or wound protectors cannot solve the problem of remote or multifocal recurrence. This is confirmed in our inquiry: in six cases of tumor seeding of carcinomas other than gallbladder and colon, the tumor was not manipulated at all during the laparoscopic procedure. Under this special condition the role of laparoscopic tumor staging with and without intraoperative ultrasound must be critically evaluated. Unfortunately, we were not able to collect data about the total number of diagnostic or therapeutic laparoscopies performed on patients with abdominal malignancies other than gallbladder and colorectal cancer in the 443 hospitals that responded, so we cannot estimate the incidence of tumor seeding of this group of oncological indications to laparoscopy.

The following aspects of laparoscopy may lead to an increased probability of wound implantation:

- Increased exfoliation of tumor cells resulting from greater manipulation near the tumor or at the tumor itself by laparoscopic instruments
- Contact between the skin incisions and malignant cells during extraction of the instruments and of the specimen
- Direct physical and chemical influence of pneumoperitoneum and pressure on tumor cell diffusion and tumor growth

Neoplastic cells circulating free in the peritoneum were demonstrated by Umpleby [37]. Recently Juhl, using immunocytological methods, found neoplastic cells in the peritoneal cavity in 27% of patients with colorectal tumors, 43% of patients with gastric cancer, and 58% of patients suffering from pancreatic cancer [38]. The same author demonstrated a relationship between the probability of the presence of tumor cells and the tumor stage. First experiments on animals seem to show a direct biologic influence from different gases on tumor cell implantation and growth in the peritoneum [38, 39].

Nontraumatic handling and retrieval of specimen in both known and nonapparent tumors, with enlargement of the extraction site whenever necessary, might perhaps reduce the risk of laparoscopic tumor seeding. The use of a cellophane bag for specimen retrieval is a logical method to avoid contact between malignant tissue and peritoneum or skin. This measure must be considered mandatory for extraction of suspected or assessed cancer tissue. Assuming that this precaution does not exclude intraperitoneal or trocar site metastatic events, and that nonapparent tumors affected only 0.35% of gallbladders in our survey and about 1% in other surgical reviews, it cannot be generally recommended during all laparoscopic cholecystectomies.

References

1. Nduka CC, Monson JRT, Menzies-Gow N, Darzi A(1994) Abdominal wall metastases following laparoscopy. Br J Surg 81:648
2. Wexner SD, Cohen SM (1995) Port site metastases after laparoscopic colorectal surgery for cure of malignancy. Br J Surg 82:295
3. Kindermann G, Maaßen V, Kuhn W (1996) Laparoscopic management of ovarian tumors subsequently diagnosed as malignant. J Pelvic Surg 2:245
4. Ballantyne GH (1995) Laparoscopic-assisted colorectal surgery: review of results in 752 patients. Gastroenterol 3:75–89
5. Lacy AM, Garcia-Valdecas JC, Pique JM et al (1995) Short-term outcome analysis of a randomized study comparing laparoscopic vs open colectomy for cancer. Surg Endosc 9:1101–1105
6. Lord SA, Larach SW, Ferrara A et al (1996) Laparoscopic resections of colorectal carcinoma. A three year experience. Dis Colon Rectum 39: 148–154
7. Hughes ES, McDermott FT, Polglase AL, Johnson WR (1983) Tumor recurrence in the abdominal wall scar tissue after large bowel cancer surgery. Dis Colon Rectum 26:571–572
8. Gunderson LL, Sosin H (1994) Areas of failure found at reoperation (second or sympto-

matic look) following – curative surgery – for adenocarcinoma of the rectum: clinicopathologic correlation and implications for adjuvant therapy. Cancer 34:1278–1292

9. Franklin ME, Rosenthal D, Norem RF (1995) Prospective evaluation of laparoscopic colon resection versus open colon resection for adenocarcinoma. Surg Endosc 9:811

10. Kwok SPY, Lau WY, Carey PD, Kelly SB, Leung Kl, Li AKC (1996) Prospective evaluation of laparoscopic-assisted large-bowel excision for cancer. Ann Surg 223:170

11. Hoffman GC, Baker JW, Doxey JB, Hubbard GW, Ruffin WK, Wishner JA (1996) Minimally invasive surgery for colorectal cancer. Initial follow-up. Ann Surg 223:790

12. Fleshman JW, Fry RD, Birnbaum EH, Kodner IJ (1996) Laparoscopic-assisted and minilaparotomy approaches to colorectal disease are similar in early outcome. Dis Colon Rectum 39:15

13. Monson JRT, Hill ADK, Darzi A (1995) Laparoscopic colonic surgery. Br J Surg 82:150

14. Wexner SD, Cohen SM, Ulrich A, Reissman P (1995) Laparoscopic colorectal surgery – Are we being honest with our patients? Dis Colon Rectum 38:723

15. Martinez J, Targarona EM, Balagué C, Pera Mi, Trias M (1995) Port site metastasis. An unresolved problem in laparoscopic surgery. A review. Int Surg 80:315

16. Fingerhut A (1995) Laparoscopic colectomy. The French experience. In: Jager R, Wexner SD (eds) Laparoscopic colorectal surgery. Churchill Livingstone, New York

17. Gleeson NC, Nicosia SV, Mark JE, Hoffmann MS, Cavanagh D (1993) Abdominal wall metastasis from ovarian cancer after laparoscopy. Am J Obstet Gyn 169:322

18. Ng JWT, Lee KKW, Chan AYT (1994) Documentation of tumor seeding complicating laparoscopic cholecystectomy for unsuspected gallbladder carcinoma. Surgery 115:530

19. Vukasin P, Ortega AE, Greene FL, Steele GD, Simons AJ, Anthone GJ, Weston LA, Beart RW (1996) Wound recurrence following laparoscopic colon cancer resection. Results of the American Society of Colon and Rectal Surgeons Laparoscopic registry. Dis Colon Rectum 39[Suppl 10]:20–2315

20. Anderson DN, Driver CP, Miller SS (1996) Port recurrence after laparoscopic surgery: The AESGBI experience (abstract). Minim Invasive Ther 5:100

21. Cook TA, Dehn TBC (1996) Port-site metastases in patients undergoing laparoscopy for gastrointestinal malignancy. Br J Surg 83:1419

22. Jones RS (1990) Carcinoma of the gallbladder. Surg Clin North Am 70:1419

23. Henson DE, Albores-Saavedra J, Corle D (1992) Carcinoma of the gallbladder. Histologic types, stage of disease, grade, and survival rates. Cancer 70:1493

24. Bergdahl L (1980) Gallbladder carcinoma first diagnosed at microscopic examination of gallbladders removed for presumed benign disease. Ann Surg 191:19

25. Shirai Y, Yoshida K, Tsukada K, Muto T (1991) Inapparent carcinoma of the gallbladder. An appraisal of a radical second operation after simple cholecystectomy. Ann Surg 215:326

26. O'Rourke N, Price PM, Kelly S, Sikora K (1993) Tumor inoculation during laparoscopy. Lancet 342:68

27. Fong Y, Brennan MF, Turnbull A, Colt DG, Blumgart LH (1993) Gallbladder cancer discovered during laparoscopic surgery. Arch Surg 128:1054

28. Pezet D, Frondinier E, Rotman N, Guy L, Lemesle P, Lointier P, Chipponi J (1992) Parietal seeding of carcinoma of the gallbladder after laparoscopic cholecystectomy. Br J Surg 79:230

29. Mouiel J, Crafa F, Cursio R, Gugenheim J (1996) Oncological risks in laparoscopic surgery. In: Paolucci V, Schaeff B (eds) Gasless laparoscopy in general surgery and gynecology. Diagnostic and therapeutic procedures. Thieme International, New York, pp 24–29

30. Prasad A, Avery C, Foley RJ (1994) Abdominal wall metastases following laparoscopy. Br J Surg 81:1697

31. Berends FJ, Kazemier G, Bonjer HJ, Lange JF (1994) Subcutaneous metastases after laparo-scopic colectomy. Lancet 344:58
32. Ramos JM, Gupta S, Anthone GJ, Ortega AE, Simons AJ, Beart RW (1994) Laparoscopy and colon cancer. Is the port site at risk? A preliminary report. Arch Surg 129:897
33. Russi EG, Pergolizzi S, Mesiti M, Rizzo M, d'Aquino A, Altavilla G, Adamo V (1992) Unusual relapse of hepatocellular carcinoma. Cancer 70:1483
34. Cava A, Roman J, Gonzales Quintela A, Martin F, Aramburo P (1990) Subcutaneous metasta-sis following laparoscopy in gastric adenocarcinoma. Eur J Surg Oncol 16:63
35. Siriwardena A, Samarji WN (1993) Cutaneous tumour seeding from a previously undiag-nosed pancreatic carcinoma after laparoscopic cholecystectomy. Ann R Coll Surg Engl 75:199
36. Nieveen van Dijkum EJM, de Wit LTh, Obertop H, Gouma DJ (1996) Port-site metastases following diagnostic laparoscopy. Br J Surg 83:1793
37. Umpleby HC, Fermor B, Symes MO, Williamson RCN (1984) Viability of exfoliated colorec-tal carcinoma cells. Br J Surg 71:859
38. Juhl H, Stritzel M, Wroblewski A (1994) Immunocytological detection of micro-metastatic cells: comparative evaluation of findings in the peritoneal and pancreatic cancer patients. Int J Cancer 57:330
39. Köckerling F, Reymond MA, Schneider C, Hohenberger W (1997) Fehler und Gefahren in der onkologischen laparoskopischen Chirurgie. Chirurg 68:215

Results and Strategies of Clinical Applications: Gastrointestinal Tract

Staging Laparoscopy for Esophageal Cancer

B. Rau · M. Hünerbein · P. Hohenberger · P.M. Schlag

Introduction

The overall 5-year survival rate of esophageal cancer even after resection with clear margins (R0 resection) ranges only between 10% and 20%, demonstrating the dismal prognosis of this disease. Controlled randomized trials suggested that combined modality therapy may improve outcome of those patients with operable disease and without distant metastases particularly following the approach of preoperative radiation plus chemotherapy [16]. In comparison, there are no convincing data from prospectively randomized trials documenting an advantage of postoperative adjuvant chemo- or radiotherapy [5].

Squamous cell cancer is the tumor type most often diagnosed, and adenocarcinoma was a rather rare disease until recent years showed increasing incidence of adenocarcinoma in the western hemisphere. There is no prognostic difference between the two tumor types. Only patients with early adenocarcinoma appear to have a survival advantage compared with patients with squamous cell carcinoma.

Patients with squamous cell cancer often suffer from alcoholic liver disease or chronic bronchitis due to heavy smoking. In contrast, adenocarcinoma often arises in people with gastroesophageal reflux disease due to decreased functioning of the lower esophageal sphincter [9]. However, this condition is often associated with the treatment of ischemic heart disease. From this point of view, the underlying medical conditions in both subtypes of esophageal cancer make a careful selection of patients mandatory whether radical resection by an abdominothoracic approach is intended or combined modality therapy is thought to be the treatment of choice.

Preoperative radiochemotherapy (RChT) was first introduced to the treatment of patients suffering from squamous cell cancer of the anus by Nigro et al. [26], and strategies were adopted from this experience to the treatment of esophageal cancer. Response rates to RChT of more than 50% and up to 20% pathological complete remissions were reported [5]. However, resection of the residual lesion may be required to avoid local recurrences. To date, there has been no general acceptance of preoperative radiochemotherapy as the standard of care. The optimum radiation field and dose as well as the ideal combination of drugs and administration schedule have yet to be defined. As a consequence, combined modality therapy is often performed under study conditions and accurate staging before entering patients into a trial is a prerequisite.

General Therapeutic Approach to Esophageal Cancer

Therapeutic preferences clearly address tumor stage: in T1 or T2 tumors with no evidence of lymphatic metastases at endosonography (uT0) or computed tomography (CT) scan, surgical resection is the treatment of first choice. In T2 or T3 lesions with nodal involvement (N+), inclusion in trials exploring surgical resection after preoperative RChT is often favored. Patients with significant comorbidity considered unfit for major surgery are often treated by RChT alone. In patients with metastatic disease, treatment is directed toward palliation of symptoms. Restoration of swallowing and relief of pain can be achieved by radio (chemo)therapy [29] and/or endoscopic treatment using self-expanding metal stents [20], laser ablation [1], intraluminal high-dose brachytherapy [33], or photodynamic treatment [23]. Palliative resection of the esophagus is indicated in selected patients only. Thus exact staging should not take place during laparotomy.

It does not make any sense to treat a patient within a protocol for neoadjuvant therapy if distant metastases are already present but remain undetected. The methods to palliate symptoms (stent placement, laser vaporization, radiotherapy, palliative surgery) are very effective and save patients' physical and emotional resources otherwise stressed during preoperative therapy. With respect to the application of radiotherapy, it must be borne in mind that preoperative regimens and palliative schedules are different. In the preoperative setting, radiation doses used range from 40 to 45 Gy. After a time interval of approximately 4 weeks, the operation follows. If metastatic disease is found during laparotomy or thoracotomy, it makes no sense to proceed (re-start) with radiation therapy to the full palliative dose of 55–60 Gy for radiobiologic reasons (time interval between irradiation series is too long). Consequently, these patients may not receive adequate treatment because they are wrongly treated within a neoadjuvant protocol initially. Therefore, an optimum of preoperative staging must be guaranteed.

What is the advantage of staging laparoscopy in patients with esophageal cancer in this setting?

- To rule out disseminated disease (peritoneal spread, liver metastases)
- To assess intra-abdominal lymph nodes (juxtaregional nodes)
- To provide additional information on the radiation field in palliative cases
- To confirm eligibility for trials, particularly preoperative combined modality therapy based on a higher degree of certainty about the stage of disease
- To insert intestinal feeding tube for preoperative treatment
- To prove whether and to what extent liver cirrhosis is present

Staging Methods and Requirements

Routine staging procedures in esophageal cancer include endoscopy, abdominal ultrasound (US), and endoluminal US as well as CT scanning of the thorax and upper abdomen. The assessment of wall infiltration of the tumor (T category) can be achieved with an accuracy of about 85% (Table 1) [12, 15].

Endoluminal US is able to improve the determination of local tumor spread and may detect peritumoral lymph node metastases (Table 2). Transesophageal

Table 1. Additional findings with staging laparoscopy compared to conventional staging including CT and US in squamous cell carcinoma

Author	Year	Patients	PER	LN	HEP	OTH	Σ
Shandall [30]	1985	23	3 (13%)	9 (39%)	4 (17%)	0	16 (70%)
Dagnini [10]	1986	280[a]	26 (9%)	10 (4%)	11 (4%)	5 (2%)	52 (19%)
Watt [34]	1989	36	4 (11%)	13 (36%)	8 (22%)	0	15 (69%)
O'Brien [27]	1995	30	0	NA	2 (7%)	3 (10%)	5 (17%)
Own results	1998	65	1 (8%)	7 (41%)	7 (41%)	0	15 (23%)

PER, peritoneal carcinomatosa; LN, lymph node metastases at M1 positions; HEP, liver metastases; OTH, others; NA, not available.
[a]Additional findings were presented at laparotomy as false negative findings in liver ($n=7$) and peritoneal spread ($n=4$) patients.

Table 2. Accuracy of detecting intra-abdominal lymph node metastases with different imaging modalities in esophageal cancer

Author	Year	LASC and/or LAPUS	US	CT
Bonavina [6]	1997	96%	82%	90%
Goletti [14]	1995	89%	60%	
Watt [34]	1989	72%	52%	57%

LASC, laparoscopy; LAPUS, laparoscopic ultrasound; US, transcutaneous ultrasound; CT, computer tomography.

biopsy of suspicious lymph nodes is a method applied at selected centers [17]. However, curability of the disease is not a problem of local spread but of regional and juxtaregional dissemination. A French trial used tumor thickness and the size of the lymph nodes (if >1 cm) as the sole criteria for stage attribution [8]. From that point of view, it is not astonishing that a considerable proportion of patients treated with maximum effort to remove the locally obstructive tumor in reality suffered from metastatic disease. Trials in esophageal cancer with the main focus on improving resectability by preoperative radiochemotherapy are looking for disease-free survival. However, a considerable number of patients already have abdominal metastases in terms of nodal spread or peritoneal carcinosis not detected by conventional imaging (Table 3). These patients are wrongly judged to be curable and subjected to preoperative radiotherapy but remain without adequate treatment for their disseminated disease. On the other hand, even if effective treatment was administered to control tumor growth locally or locoregionally these efforts may be overridden by tumor dissemination outside the therapeutic focus. These patients often undergo abdominothoracic resection in a metastatic stage of disease with poor postoperative survival [2]. Hence, esophageal cancer is a type of tumor requiring the utmost diagnostic accuracy to allocate patients to adequate treatment regimens.

Table 3. Accuracy of detecting liver metastases with different imaging modalities in esophageal cancer

Author	Year	LASC and/or LAPUS	US	CT
Bonavina [6]	1997	98%	98%	98%
Goletti [14]	1995	100%		76%
Watt [34]	1989	96%	83%	85%
Shandall [30]	1985	96%	76%	

LASC, laparoscopy; LAPUS, laparoscopic ultrasound; US, transcutaneous ultrasound; CT, computer tomography.

Table 4. Accuracy of detecting intra-abdominal peritoneal tumor spread with different imaging modalities in esophageal cancer

Author	Year	LASC and/or LAPUS	US	CT
Bonavina [6]	1997	96%	88%	88%
Watt [34]	1989	98%	89%	–

LASC, laparoscopy; LAPUS, laparoscopic ultrasound; US, transcutaneous ultrasound; CT, computer tomography.

The results of attempts to detect distant metastases (M category) preoperatively by means of radiological imaging remain disappointing (Table 4). Prospectively documented comparative studies revealed the limitations of transcutaneous ultrasonography and CT scans in small-volume metastastic disease of the liver as well as in detecting peritoneal tumor spread [28].

Operative Technique of Staging Laparoscopy for Esophageal Cancer

Staging laparoscopy is performed under general anesthesia. After the incision line intended for subsequent laparotomy is indicated, carbon dioxide is insufflated through a Veress needle into the abdominal cavity until a pressure of 12–15 mmHg is reached. After removal of the needle, a 10-mm trocar for the 45° side-viewing optic is inserted. Whenever possible, the trocar is placed into the linea alba around the umbilicus depending on the body shape. In the case of previous surgery in this area, another place should be found without adhesions expected or the Hasson approach can be used (see page 22). Additional trocars are introduced following the scheme shown in Fig. 1. With this arrangement of trocars almost every intra-abdominal space can be explored. Also, palliative laparoscopic procedures (gastro-entero-anastomosis, placement of feeding tubes) can be performed.

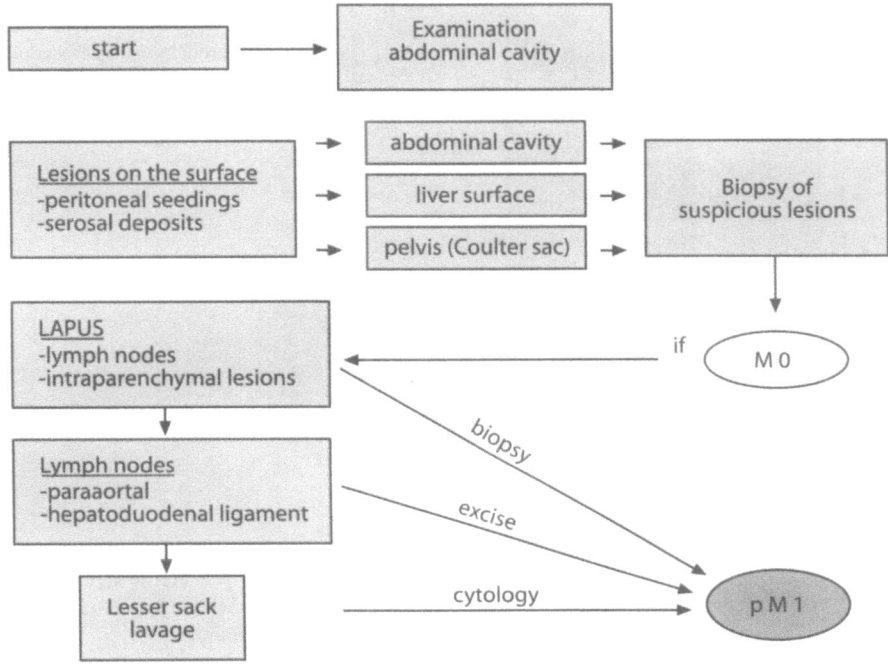

Fig. 1. Algorithm of staging laparoscopy (*LAPUS*, laparoscopic ultrasound)

The Sequence of Explorative Steps

1. Careful examination of the abdominal cavity is performed with respect to free fluid, peritoneal and serosal deposits, and lesions on the surface of the liver.
2. A second trocar (usually 5 mm) is placed in the epigastric angle to elevate the left liver lobe for examination of the infrahepatic space, the esophagogastric junction, and the hepatoduodenal ligament with attention to enlarged lymph nodes. If the size and/or weight of the left liver is too great or the anatomical conditions of the liver and the upper abdominal quadrant can withstand the use of a stab, a fan-shaped retractor can be inserted after changing the 5-mm trocar to 10-mm equipment.
3. Lesser sac exploration can be performed by two ways: via the minor omentum or by dividing the gastrocolic ligament. In case of performing the latter approach, two additional trocars are required and are placed at the anterior axillary line of the mid or upper abdominal quadrant. These trocar insertions are to be excised and used as drainage canals during subsequent laparotomy.
4. With the placement of all these trocars, exploration of the Coulter sac by eventration is rather simple. The Trendelenburg position is very helpful to move the small bowel from the pelvis to the mid and upper part of the abdominal cavity.

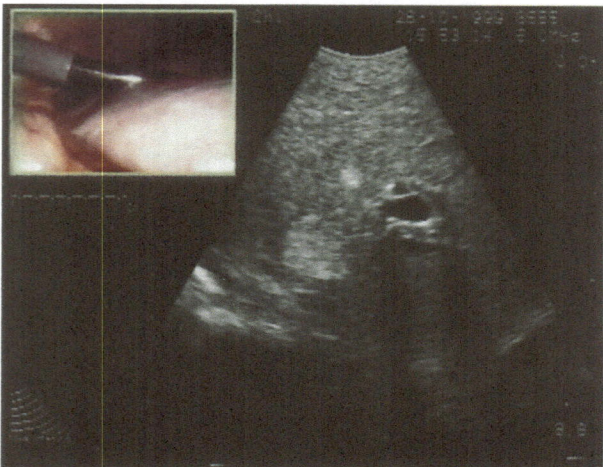

Fig. 2. Small metastases located deeply in the liver parenchyma laparoscopic ultrasound is helpful in discrimination from he-mangioma

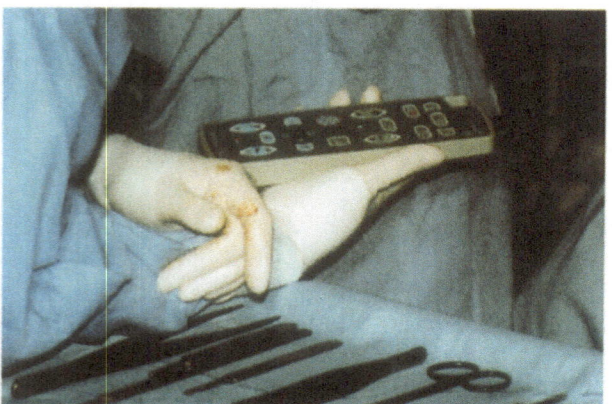

Fig. 3. Sterile hand equipment, to handle ultrasound

5. If there are no signs of metastatic spread on laparoscopy, the next step is to insert a flexible probe for laparoscopic US (e.g., B&K type 9130). The US probe is introduced through a 10-mm trocar usually on the right side of the abdomen (see also chapter by Hünerbein et al., this volume). US application focuses on intraparenchymal lesions of the liver or suspicious lymph nodes at metastatic (M1) positions such as para-aortal or at the hepatoduodenal ligament (Fig. 2 and 3).

6. Suspicious lymph nodes are excised with caution for adjacent vessels and sent for frozen section (Fig. 4). Intraparenchymal lesions of the liver may be approached sometimes with more difficulty. True-cut needle biopsies can be taken under optical and ultrasonographic guidance.

Fig. 4. Transgastric laparoscopic ultrasound in esophageal cancer demonstrating enlarged lymph nodes at the celiac axis. Doppler ultrasound is helpful for exact localisation and to avoid bleeding during excisional lymph node tiopsy

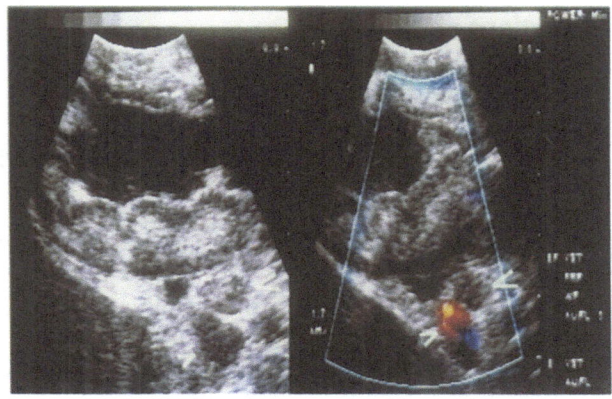

If metastatic disease is detected during laparoscopic staging, the procedure can be continued with palliative surgery. If conversion to laparotomy is necessary, all trocar positions will be part of the incision line or used for insertion of drains.

If the insertion of a feeding tube (e.g., Freka-PEG Universal-Intestinal-Set, Germany, Bad Homburg; or COMPAT Jejunalcath, Germany Wander GmbH, Celle) seems reasonable during preoperative radiotherapy, this can be performed through a separate incision. The stomach or jejunal wall is perforated, and the tube placed under laparoscopic vision and afterwards fixed with resorbable sutures.

In our clinical routine, laparoscopy and definitive surgery is not performed on the same day for the following reasons:

- Additional information obtained during laparoscopy may open new treatment options
- Histological confirmation of frozen tissue examination results must be awaited
- A definitive decision must be made as to whether operation alone or a multimodal therapeutic concept is the treatment of choice
- Informed consent must be obtained from the patient on the basis of all available information
- Operating room capacity can be planned more exactly
- However, if the decision tree is agreed to by the patient before operation, laparoscopy can be converted into open laparotomy. Laparoscopic preparation can be extended, for example, by converting of the stomach to a tube for esophageal replacement. Mobilizing of the duodenum can also be performed laparoscopically, and esophageal resection by thoracotomy will be the only step done by open surgery.

Regions of Interest

Assessment of Resectability

Local tumor extension of esophageal cancer of the upper third tends to involve the trachea, whereas tumors of the middle third may invade to the aorta, tracheal bifurcation, or main stem bronchi. Tumors of the lower third of the esophagus are close to the descending aorta, the vertebral fascia, and the diaphragm, and those tissues are at risk of infiltration. All anatomical compartments mentioned cannot be explored by laparoscopy, and endoluminal US best determines the extent of tumor invasion [12, 15].

Thoracoscopy, especially when combined with endoluminal US, might be useful to assess resectability in tumors localized in the mid third of the esophagus as well as invasion to the pleura and pericardium. With subsequent thoracoscopic esophageal resection, 4 of 22 patients (18%) required conversion to thoracotomy [24]. Whether tumors are fixed by true malignant invasion or because of peritumorous inflammation cannot be examined exactly with endoscopical means, particularly in patients with preexisting diseases such as chronic bronchitis or enlarged lymph nodes after tuberculosis. Esophageal cancer of the distal third, especially when infiltrating the region of the cardia, may be approached by laparoscopy. Infiltration of the diaphragm is visible and can be biopsied by laparoscopic view after division of the lesser omentum.

Assessment of Visuable Lesions

Peritoneal Spread

Peritoneal carcinomatosis in squamous cell carcinoma of the esophagus is rare. During staging laparoscopy, Watt and coworkers in 4 of 19 patients revealed peritoneal carcinomatosis that had not been detected by conventional imaging (CT scan, US). Our results also demonstrated a very small number of patients with peritoneal seedings. O'Brien and colleagues did not find any peritoneal metastasis in 30 patients with squamous cell cancer [27].

In order not to miss small peritoneal lesions, exploration of the abdominal cavity must include all parts of the surface of the liver, the upper abdominal peritoneal surface, the Coulter sac after displacing the small bowel, and the lesser sac in distal esophageal cancer.

Staging laparoscopy is a sensitive and specific method to detect peritoneal tumor dissemination. Diagnostic accuracy by imaging techniques such as CT and transcutaneous US are limited. Lesions smaller than 1 cm in diameter are rarely detected and are usually missed unless indirect signs such as ascites are present.

Bonavina and colleagues demonstrated that laparoscopy showed a higher sensitivity than US and CT in detecting peritoneal metastases (71% vs. 14% in each of the other modalities) [6]. Similar results were reported by Watt and Shandall, who showed an accuracy of 89% with US compared with 98% with laparoscopy. In just one patient a lesion detected during open laparotomy was missed laparoscopically but was located at the inferior surface of the transverse mesocolon [34].

Assessment of Nonvisuable Lesions

Lymph Node Metastases

The prognostic value of lymph node metastases in esophageal cancer has been well described [3, 22]. In upper esophageal cancer, lymph node metastases occur predominantly in the cervical region including the supraclavicular nodes, whereas for the intrathoracic esophagus the mediastinal, paracardial, and upper perigastric nodes belong to the regional spread. Celiac axis nodes can be called regional only in cancer of the lower esophagus.

Cervical lymph node metastases, present in up to 31% of patients, are correctly detected by US in 88% of patients [25]. Regarding intrathoracic nodes, a prospective, multiinstitutional study demonstrated that thoracoscopy accurately detected their status in 28 of 30 patients (93%) [19]. However, mediastinal lymph nodes belong to the regional lymph nodes and are included in a mono bloc resection [11].

All lymph nodes localized para-aortally or in the hepatoduodenal ligament are classified as distant metastases according to the UICC [31]. Involvement of celiac nodes (M1-LYM) occurs in 10% of the esophagus cancer located in the cervical region and up to 44% in patients with mid-third tumors. Consequently, laparoscopy must focus on these regions, using laparoscopic US as an essential tool. In our series, lymph node metastases (M1-LYM) were the most frequent site of metastatic spread not known before laparoscopy from conventional imaging findings (41% of the cases).

Stell and coworkers [32] reported superior accuracy of laparoscopy in predicting intra-abdominal lymph nodes occupied by tumor with 65% compared with percutaneous US with 34% or CT with 45%. In another series, laparoscopy also showed a higher sensitivity than US and CT in detecting nodal metastases (78% vs. 11% vs. 55%, respectively) [6]. Krasna and coworkers demonstrated a diagnostic accuracy in detecting lymph node metastases in 94%, when staging used a combined thoracoscopic and laparoscopic approach [18].

Liver

The frequency of liver metastases depends on the localization of the primary tumor. Autopsy findings revealed liver metastases in 16% of upper third tumors, 29% of mid-third tumors, and 43% of tumor of the distal third of the esophagus [7]. A prospective comparison of laparoscopy and combined imaging (CT and US) in the preoperative staging of distal esophageal and gastric cancer in patients who were selected for surgery was carried out by O'Brien and coworkers, who reported an incidence of metastatic disease in 27% of patients. In the overall picture, metastases were detected by laparoscopy with a sensitivity of 77% whereas combined imaging procedures reached a sensitivity of only 38%. Concerning liv-

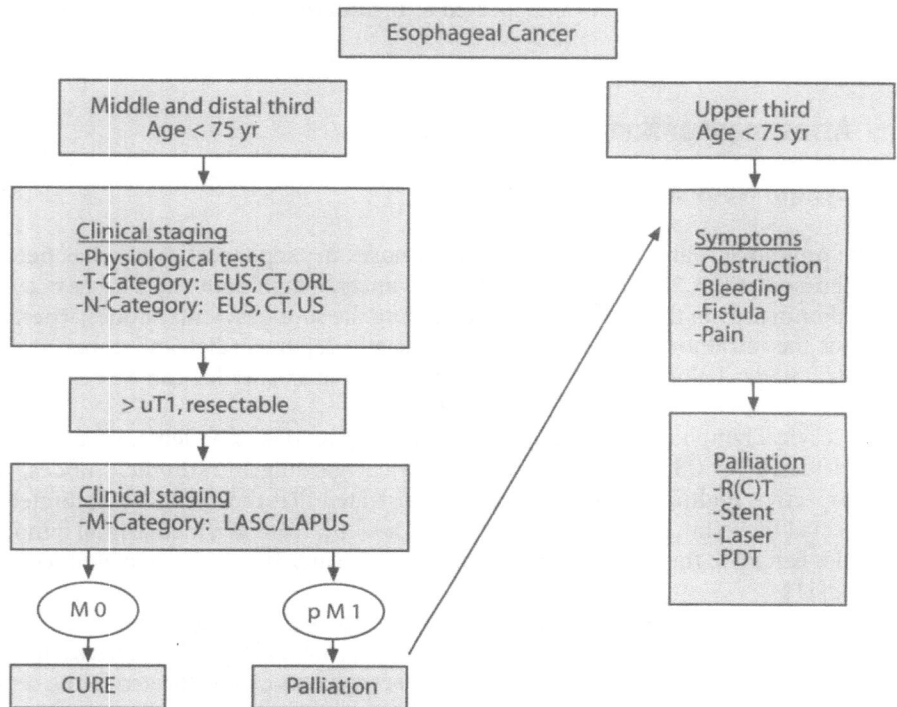

Fig. 5. Algorithm of surgical decisions in the management of esophageal cancer. Abbreviations: *EUS*, endorectal ultrasound; *ORL*, otorhinolaryngology; *LASC*, laparoscopy; *LAPUS*, laparoscopic ultrasound; *R(C)T*, radio-(chemo)-therapy; *PDT*, photodynamic therapy

er metastases, laparoscopy demonstrated a sensitivity of 60% in comparison to combined imaging showing a sensitivity of 47% [27]. Similar data were presented by Bonavina et al. with a sensitivity to detect liver metastases by laparoscopy in 86% compared to US and CT with 71%, respectively [6].

In our experience, in 7 of 17 patients (41%) with esophageal cancer, liver metastases not known from imaging findings could be detected by laparoscopy. In another patient, liver metastases were detected by laparoscopic US. The overall proportion of patients with new information concerning tumor spread after staging laparoscopy added up to 21%. Disseminated disease was not found in early cancer (T1 lesions). The greater the depth of tumor infiltration the higher the percentage of lesions detected additionally: in 2 out of 10 uT2 tumors (20%) and in 10 out of 39 uT3-tumors (26%), we found tumor spread during staging laparoscopy previously unknown.

Improvement of the treatment of esophageal cancer begins with a precise staging, and beyond laparoscopy including US no better tools seem to be available.

It should not be disregarded that some authors found that laparoscopy and laparoscopic ultrasonography was not an effective staging technique for squamous cell carcinoma of the middle and lower esophagus and particularly estimated the inclusion of laparoscopic ultrasonography seemed to be of little benefit [4, 28]. This might be due to the low patient numbers assessed and due to the fact that tumors with low risk for disseminated disease were selected.

Preliminary reports on the use of positron emission tomography (PET) in patients with esophageal cancer showed a sensitivity of 88%, a specificity of 93%, and accuracy of 91% for the detection of distant metastases. For locoregional nodal metastases, the sensitivity was 45%, the specificity was 100%, and the accuracy was 48% [21]. In another study, the results of PET changed clinical management in 17% of patients [13]. Further studies will have to be awaited before including PET in the staging of spread outside the abdominal cavity. Laparoscopy improves the accuracy of clinical staging and is an integral part of the decision-making process in esophageal cancer (Fig. 5).

References

1. Adam A, Ellul J, Watkinson AF, Tan BS, Morgan RA, Saunders MP, Mason RC (1997) Palliation of inoperable esophageal carcinoma: a prospective randomized trial of laser therapy and stent placement. Radiology 202:344–348
2. Alcantara PSM, Spencer-Netto FAC, Silva-Junior JF, Soares LA, Pollara WM, Bevilacqua RG (1997) Gastro-esophageal isoperistaltic bypass in the palliation of irresectable thoracic esophageal cancer. Int Surg 82:249–253
3. Baba M, Aikou T, Yoshinaka H, Natsugoe S, Fukumoto T, Shimazu H, Akazawa K (1994) Long-term results of subtotal esophagectomy with three-field lymphadenectomy for carcinoma of the esophagus. Ann Surg 219:310–316
4. Bemelman WA, de Wit LT, van Delden OM, Smits NJ, Obertop H, Rauws EJ, Gouma DJ (1995) Diagnostic laparoscopy combined with laparoscopic ultrasonography in staging of cancer of the pancreatic head region. Br J Surg 82:820–824
5. Benhidjeb T, Hohenberger P (2001) Cancer of the esophagus. In: Souhami R, Tannock I, Hohenberger P, Horiot JC (eds). Oxford Textbook of Oncology. Oxford University Press
6. Bonavina L, Incarbone R, Lattuada E, Segalin A, Cesana B, Peracchia A (1997) Preoperative laparoscopy in management of patients with carcinoma of the esophagus and of the esophagogastric junction. J Surg Oncol 65:171–174
7. Bosch A, Frias Z, Caldwell WL, Jaeschke WH (1979) Autopsy findings in carcinoma of the oesophagus. Acta Radiol Oncol 18:103–106
8. Bosset JF, Gignoux M, Triboulet JP, et al (1997) Chemoradiotherapy followed by surgery compared with surgery alone in squamous cell cancer of the esophagus. N Engl J Med 337:161–167
9. Coenraad M, Masclee AA, Straathof JW, et al (1998) Is Barrett's esophagus characterized by more pronounced acid reflux than severe esophagitis? Am J Gastroenterol 93:108–172
10. Dagnini G, Caldironi MW, Marin G, Buzzaccarini O, Tremolada C, Ruol A (1986) Laparoscopy in abdominal staging of esophageal carcinoma. Gastrointest Endosc 32:400–402
11. DeMeester TR, Barlow AP (1988) Surgery and current management for cancer of the esophagus and cardia. Curr Probl Surg 12:241–327
12. Dittler HJ, Siewert JR (1993) Role of endoscopic ultrasonography in esophageal carcinoma. Endoscopy 25:156–161

13. Flanagan FL, Dehdashti F, Giegel BA, et al (1997) Staging of esophageal cancer with 18F-Fluorodeoxyglucose positron emission tomography. AJR 168:417–424

14. Goletti O, Buccianti P, Chiarugi M, Pieri L, Sbragia P, Cavina E (19995) Laparoscopic sonography in screening metastases from gastrointestinal cancer: comparative accuracy with traditional procedures. Surg Laparosc Endosc 5:176–182

15. Grimm H, Binmoeller KF, Hamper K, Koch J, Henne-Bruns D, Soehendra N (1993) Endosonography for preoperative locoregional staging of esophageal and gastric cancer. Endoscopy 25:224–230

16. Herskovic A, Martz K, al-Sarraf M, et al (1992) Combined chemotherapy and radiotherapy compared with radiotherapy alone in patients with cancer of the esophagus. N Engl J Med 326:1593–1598

17. Hünerbein M, Totkas S, Balanou P, Handke T, Schlag PM (1999) EUS-guided fine needle biopsy: minimally invasive access to metastatic or recurrent cancer. Eur J Ultrasound 10:151–157

18. Krasna MJ (1995) Thoracoscopic staging of esophageal carcinoma. Chest Surg Clin N Am 5:489–513

19. Krasna MJ (1998) Advances in staging of esophageal carcinoma. Chest 113:107S–111S

20. Ludwig D, Dehne A, Burmester E, Wiedemann GJ, Stange EF (1998) Treatment of unresectable carcinoma of the esophagus or the gastroesophageal junction by mesh stents with or without radiochemotherapy. Int J Oncol 13:583–588

21. Luketich JD, Schauer PR, Meltzer CC, et al (1997) Role of positron emission tomography in staging esophageal cancer. Ann Thorac Surg 64:765–769

22. Matsubara T, Ueda M, Nakajima T (1995) Preoperative assessment of lymph nodes in the prediction of disease spread and outcome in cancer of the thoracic oesophagus. Br J Surg 82:356–359

23. McCaughan JS Jr, Ellison EC, Guy JT, Hicks WJ, Jones JJ, Laufman LR, May E, Nims TA, Spiridonidis CH, Williams TE (1996) Photodynamic therapy for esophageal malignancy: a prospective twelve-year study. Ann Thorac Surg 62:1005–1009

24. Mortensen MB, Scheel Hincke JD, Madsen MR, Qvist N, Hovendal C (1996) Combined endoscopic ultrasonography and laparoscopic ultrasonography in the pretherapeutic assessment of resectability in patients with upper gastrointestinal malignancies. Scand J Gastroenterol 31:1115–1119

25. Natsugoe S, Yoshinaka H, Shimada M, Shirao K, Nakano S, Kusano C, Baba M, Fukumoto T, Takao S, Aikou T (1999) Assessment of cervical lymph node metastasis in esophageal carcinoma using ultrasonography. Ann Surg 229:62–66

26. Nigro ND, Seydel HG, Considine B, Vaitkevicius VK, Leichman L et al (1983) Combined preoperative radiation and chemotherapy for squamous cell carcinoma of the anal canal. Cancer 51:1826

27. O'Brien MG, Fitzgerald EF, Lee G, Crowley M, Shanahan F, O'Sullivan GC (1995) A prospective comparison of laparoscopy and imaging in the staging of esophagogastric cancer before surgery. Am J Gastroenterol 90:2191–2194

28. Romijn MG, van Overhagen H, Spillenaar Bilgen EJ, Ijzermans JN, Tilanus HW, Lameris JS (1998) Laparoscopy and laparoscopic ultrasonography in staging of oesophageal and cardial carcinoma. Br J Surg 85:1010–1012

29. Seitz JF, Giovannini M, Padaut Cesana J, Fuentes P, Giudicelli R, Gauthier AP, Carcassonne Y (1990) Inoperable nonmetastatic squamous cell carcinoma of the esophagus managed by concomitant chemotherapy (5-fluorouracil and cisplatin) and radiation therapy. Cancer 66:214–219

30. Shandall A, Johnson C (1985) Laparoscopy or scanning in oesophageal and gastric carcinoma? Br J Surg 72:449–451

31. Sobin LH, Wittekind C (1997) TNM classification of malignant tumours. Wiley-Liss, New York Chichester Weinheim Brisbane Singapore Toronto
32. Stell DA, Carter CR, Stewart I, Anderson JR (1996) Prospective comparison of laparoscopy, ultrasonography and computed tomography in the staging of gastric cancer. Br J Surg 83:1260–1262
33. Taal BG, Aleman BM, Koning CC, Boot H (1996) High dose rate brachytherapy before external beam irradiation in inoperable oesophageal cancer. Br J Cancer 74:1452–1457
34. Watt I, Stewart I, Anderson D, Bell G, Anderson JR (1989) Laparoscopy, ultrasound and computed tomography in cancer of the oesophagus and gastric cardia: a prospective comparison for detecting intra-abdominal metastases. Br J Surg 76:1036–1039

The Role of Laparoscopy in the Staging of Gastric Cancer

J.B. Koea · M.S. Karpeh

Introduction

The earliest recorded use of laparoscopy in patients with carcinoma of the stomach is from 1971 [1], when it was used to provide a minimally invasive means of diagnosing intra-abdominal metastatic disease. Since this report a further 15 series describing its use in gastric and distal esophageal carcinoma [2–16] have been published. The use of this technique to define metastatic disease was encouraged by the observation that gastric resection in patients with metastatic disease was associated with a complication rate of 23% and a perioperative mortality rate of up to 25% [18–20]. In addition, a feature of the biology of gastric carcinoma is transperitoneal spread characteristically leaving multiple small peritoneal implants that are often not detected preoperatively. The introduction of laparoscopy expressed the recognition that the available modalities for preoperatively staging gastric cancer, namely clinical examination, plain abdominal X-ray, liver function tests, transabdominal ultrasound (US), and computed tomographic (CT) scanning were limited in their ability to define both peritoneal and hepatic metastatic disease [5] and that the performance of palliative gastric resections leaving behind residual peritoneal or hepatic metastases did not improve survival over that observed in unresected patients [19, 20].

Further impetus to the use of laparoscopy has recently been provided by the introduction of preoperative adjuvant chemotherapy in patients with advanced local (T3 or T4) disease. Initial investigations have shown that, in comparison to postoperative treatment, preoperative chemotherapy is associated with an increased rate of tumor response, resulting in an increase in resectability rate and possibly in survival [21]. Therefore, laparoscopy can now play a pivotal role in the management of gastric cancer by accurately defining those patients who are suitable for immediate gastric resection and lymphadenectomy or patients with advanced local disease who may benefit from preoperative neoadjuvant chemotherapy. In addition, M1 patients can be identified and entered into phase I or II chemotherapy protocols.

This chapter reviews the technique, results, and limitations of laparoscopy in the management of cancers of the lower esophagus/gastroesophageal junction and in cancers of the distal stomach.

Technique

Although laparoscopy has been performed under local anesthesia with discharge later the same day [5], laparoscopic examination should ideally be performed under general anesthesia because this permits peritoneal dissection and visceral manipulation. It is noteworthy that many of the reported failures of this technique to accurately stage gastric cancer occurred in patients in whom adequate adhesiolysis was not performed or thorough examination of the bowel or lesser sac was omitted [1, 4, 5].

With the patient supine and using an open technique, a 12-mm Hasson cannula is inserted into the abdominal cavity under direct vision. Intra-abdominal examination is carried out using a 30-degree angled scope. A 10-mm port can be placed in the right upper quadrant for the purposes of peritoneal lavage and biopsy. If laparoscopic ultrasound (LUS) is available, this can be directed toward the liver and the stomach. A 5- or 10-mm port can be added in the left upper quadrant for retraction and biopsy. Before undertaking formal staging any ascitic fluid should be aspirated and sent for cytology. Two hundred milliliters of normal saline should then be instilled and specimens for cytology aspirated from the pelvis and subphrenic spaces bilaterally. If present, peritoneal adhesions should then be divided and a thorough, systematic examination of the peritoneal cavity carried out. This should begin by examining the parietal peritoneum over the hemidiaphragms, anterior abdominal wall, and pelvis for metastatic disease. With the patient in 30 degrees of reverse Trendelenberg and 10 degrees of left lateral tilt, both anterior and posterior surfaces of the left lobe of the liver and anterior and inferior surfaces of the right lobe can be directly visualized. It is also possible to perform bimanual palpation of the liver with a grasping forceps inserted via the 5-mm port. Identification of deeply placed hepatic lesions can be undertaken with LUS using a 7.5-MHz probe inserted via the right upper quadrant port.

The transverse colon should then be elevated and the inferior surface of the transverse mesocolon inspected. An assessment of nodal disease along root of the mesentery and the ligament of Treitz is then carried out. The small intestine and its mesentery should then be inspected for metastases. Peritoneal or liver biopsies should be taken at this point and sent for frozen section examination. An assessment should be made of the mobility of the stomach and direct extension of disease to liver, spleen, colon, or duodenum. The lesser sac should be opened by incising the gastrohepatic ligament. This permits assessment of the mobility of the posterior gastric wall upon the peritoneum anterior to the pancreas. In addition, it is possible to assess nodal status along the left gastric vessels although it is not routine to biopsy these nodes because the presence of metastases is not the primary determinant of resectability.

At the end of the procedure the umbilical port site and the 10-mm port site should be closed with absorbable sutures to close the underlying fascia and subcuticular sutures to the skin.

Variations in technique will be defined by clinician preference and the results of preoperative discussion with the patient. In general, a negative examination is immediately followed by definitive resectional surgery under the same general anesthetic. In those patients who have metastatic disease it has been our practice to start chemotherapy and re-laparoscope to assess the response.

Results

The effectiveness of laparoscopic staging in gastric carcinoma has never been the focus of a double-blinded, prospective, randomized trial; however, a number of clinical series have clarified its role. Some of these reports include patients with either primary gastric or esophageal tumors (both adenocarcinoma and squamous cell carcinoma; e.g., [3]), and there are a number of variations in technique that make direct comparison of these series problematic. However, despite these issues a number of observations can be made.

Hospital Stay, Morbidity, and Mortality

One incidental death has been reported from a perforated sigmoid diverticulum 6 days after laparoscopic staging of a gastric cancer [6], and the same investigators reported an inadvertent cystostomy [6], although it is not clear whether this patient was catheterized or voided immediately before the procedure. Gross [2] reported one perforation of the transverse colon after the use of the Verress needle, a technique that is no longer widely used. Burke et al. [8] reported a 1% incidence of complications in 24 patients with metastatic disease after laparoscopy in comparison to an 8% complication rate in a similar group of patients staged with laparotomy only. Mean hospital stay was also lower in those patients staged with laparoscopy only (1.4 days) in comparison to those staged with laparotomy (6.8 days). This indicates that laparoscopy is a safe technique associated with a lower complication rate and a shorter hospital stay than those observed after laparotomy.

Economic Considerations

The use of laparoscopy before resection has been criticized on the basis of increased expense, and there has been no cost analysis of laparoscopy in gastric cancer. However, a prospective study of laparoscopy before resection in pancreatic carcinoma demonstrated that the introduction of laparoscopic staging (using reusable instruments) before pancreatectomy was associated with a 25% reduction in hospital charges. This was shown to result from a significant number of patients with metastatic disease avoiding an unnecessary laparotomy and the economic saving resulted from an overall decrease in hospital stay and in patient-related expenses [22].

The following sections will consider the role of laparoscopy in the staging of gastric carcinomas using the TNM system introduced by the UICC [23] and will compare these results with the other staging modalities that are currently available. Carcinomas involving the distal esophagus and gastroesophageal junction and carcinomas that affect the distal stomach are considered separately because the pathology and management issues pertaining to these tumors are different and consequently laparoscopy fulfills a slightly different role in each.

Distal Esophagus and Gastroesophageal Junction

T Stage (category)

Laparoscopy has not been used to define T stage in lesions of the distal esophagus because of their primarily mediastinal location, and endoscopic ultrasound (EUS) has rapidly become established as the method of choice. Tio et al. [24] were able to compare the results of staging with EUS in 83 patients with distal esophageal or gastroesophageal junction carcinoma with definitive pathological staging. The overall accuracy of this examination in T staging was 90%, with 6% of cases overstaged because of inflammatory change in ulcerated lesions or radiation or previous biopsy distorting the layers of the esophageal wall. Understaging occurred in 4% of cases and was due to luminal stenosis limiting the quality of the examination.

Ziegler et al. [25] assessed the accuracy of CT scan and EUS in distal esophageal carcinoma and compared both modalities to definitive pathological staging. CT scan was unable to consistently distinguish between tumors that are limited to the esophageal wall (T2) and those that extend beyond it (T3). This is a crucial issue, because there are studies underway evaluating whether patients with T2/T3 disease may benefit from preoperative chemotherapy whereas those with T1 lesions are best treated with primary resection [22]. Consequently, EUS is the method of choice for determining T stage in carcinoma of the distal esophagus.

N Stage (category)

Bonavina et al. [9] assessed the effectiveness of laparoscopy in defining celiac nodal disease in 50 patients with esophageal or gastroesophageal junction cancer. Two patients with microscopic involvement of celiac nodes were missed on laparoscopy, but overall the procedure correctly defined 7 patients with celiac metastases and 41 patients without metastatic disease. In comparison, spiral CT scanning had a 8% false negative rate and transabdominal US a 16% false negative rate and each imaging modality had a 2% false positive rate. Using a definition of malignant adenopathy as being lymph nodes of greater than 10 mm in diameter, Ziegler et al. [25] found that CT scan correctly demonstrated involved lymph nodes in 10 of 25 patients. with 15 false negatives and 3 false positives, and had an overall accuracy of 51%.

Krasna et al. [12] reported the combination of bilateral thoracoscopic staging in addition to laparoscopy in the nodal staging of patients with esophageal cancer. In 19 patients who underwent laparoscopic staging, 6 patients had involved celiac lymph nodes and 13 showed no involvement of celiac nodes. Of the 30 patients in whom the results of thoracoscopic staging could be correlated with definitive pathology, 2 of 28 patients with thoracoscopic N0 disease were found to have pathological N1 disease. Of the two patients who had N1 disease at thoracoscopic staging, one was found to be N0 and the other N1. In addition, two further patients were found to have pulmonary metastases at the time of thoracoscopy and no nodal staging was undertaken.

In comparison, EUS correctly diagnosed lymph node metastases in 60 of 64 patients with distal esophageal/gastroesophageal junction cancer, with the criteria of lymph nodes of any size with hypoechoic patterns and clearly delineated boundaries and direct extension of primary tumor to adjacent lymph nodes indicating malignant involvement [24]. There was one false negative diagnosis, and in three patients no diagnosis could be made because of esophageal stenosis. The overall accuracy of EUS in correctly staging lymph node disease was 82% [24].

M Stage (category)

Peritoneal Metastases

Bonavina et al. [9] showed that laparoscopy is extremely accurate in defining peritoneal carcinomatosis with 5 true positives, 43 true negatives, and 2 false negative examinations in 50 patients with proximal gastric or distal esophageal cancer. In comparison, both CT scan and transabdominal US had a 12% false negative rate for peritoneal carcinomatosis that was directly related to the size of the deposits, with small lesions (<10 mm in diameter) being difficult to image. Similarly, O'Brien et al. [13] found that laparoscopy defined 23 of 24 patients with proximal gastric or esophageal cancer as having peritoneal metastases. Dagnini et al. [10] described the use of laparoscopy in 371 patients with esophageal or gastroesophageal junction cancer and found that 14% of patients with primary esophageal cancers have abdominal metastases (either in celiac nodes or peritoneal disease), with the incidence increasing with more distally placed lesions. Two percent of peritoneal metastases were overlooked laparoscopically, and in general these were usually very small deposits located in the omentum or on the mesentery of the small bowel. Other investigators have found similar results [5, 9, 12].

Hepatic Metastases

Watt et al. [4] prospectively studied the accuracy of laparoscopy, transabdominal US, and CT scanning in patients with esophageal and proximal gastric cancer. Laparoscopy identified 22 of 25 hepatic metastases. There were three false negative examinations; two were due to extensive adhesions preventing thorough assessment of the liver and 1 was due to the posterior location of the deposits. In comparison, US identified 12 of these metastases, with 13 false negatives and 2 false positives. CT identified 14 hepatic metastases, with 11 false negatives and 2 false positives, and laparoscopy was significantly more sensitive than either CT scan or US [3]. However, O'Brien et al. [13] found that when newer-generation spiral CT was used, laparoscopy and CT were similar in their abilities to detect hepatic metastases (9/14 patients and 7/14 patients, respectively). Bonavina et al. [9] showed that laparoscopy, transabdominal US, and CT scan were all accurate in defining hepatic metastases, with both laparoscopy and US having a false negative rate of 2% whereas CT had a false negative rate of 4%. Laparoscopy and US each missed one hepatic lesion lying high in the right lobe, whereas CT scan missed two liver metastases.

The addition of LUS to laparoscopy may increase the accuracy of this examination in diagnosing hepatic metastases. Stein et al. [29] found that LUS diagnosed 16 hepatic metastases in 127 patients with normal abdominal US and CT scan. These investigators also found that unsuspected liver metastases were more common in patients with adenocarcinoma (up to 25% of T3/T4 patients) than in patients with squamous cell carcinoma (8% of T3/T4 patients).

Distal Cancers

Resectability

Accurate assessment of primary tumor characteristics via the laparoscope is difficult, and in five reported [3, 5–8] series this issue was not addressed and the procedure was restricted to the definition of metastatic disease only. Laparoscopic characteristics of the primary tumor suggesting unresectability are tumor immobility and adherence, particularly posteriorly with obliteration of the lesser sac, and direct invasion of the pancreas. Tumor adherence is difficult to assess and relies on demonstrating gastric mobility with forceps, opening the lesser sac via the gastrocolic or gastrohepatic ligaments, and elevating the posterior gastric wall off the surface of the pancreas. LUS has proved to be useful in this situation [28].

Three series have addressed the issue of resectability of the primary tumor. Posik et al. [1] assessed tumor fixity in 255 patients and accurately defined unresectability in 56 but had a false negative rate of 14.5% and a false positive rate of 4%. These investigators did not routinely open the lesser sac to clarify the state of the posterior plane, which limited the accuracy of their examination, and extension of disease into the pancreas was the primary cause of a false negative examination. Similarly, Kriplani et al. [5] found that if laparoscopic examination included an attempt to elevate tumor from the pancreas, then unresectability was accurately predicted in 11 of 40 patients. In contrast, Gross et al. [2] found that laparoscopy was poorly predictive of fixity and missed 2 from 46 tumors that were unresectable; however, in their hands, posterior extent of disease was not specifically addressed through the laparoscope.

T Stage (category)

Finch et al. [28] reported the addition of LUS to routine laparoscopy in the assessment of T stage. These investigators found that LUS improved the accuracy of laparoscopy alone by accurately detecting gastric wall penetration in 14 of 17 tumors thought to be resectable by laparoscopic assessment alone. LUS upstaged three patients by defining more advanced local disease in two patients and extragastric spread in one. Significantly, no patient's tumor was overstaged with LUS. However, Karpeh et al. [14] demonstrated that LUS is most accurate in defining T3 lesions and tended to overstage T1 and T2 disease. Using spiral CT scan, Davies et al. [17] were able to compare staging with CT to pathological staging in 105 patients with gastric cancer. These investigators found that CT correctly localized the site of the gastric tumor in 66% of patients, whereas the tumor was incorrectly localized in 8 patients and not seen in 25 patients, half of whom had early gastric cancer [26].

Tio et al. [24] were able to compare the results of staging with EUS to definitive pathological staging in 76 patients with gastric carcinoma. Overall, the accuracy of EUS was 83% with understaging occurring in 8%, because of luminal stenosis, and overstaging occurring in 9%, because of inflammatory changes in the gastric wall.

N Stage (category)

Laparoscopy has not been extensively utilized in the assessment of lymph node disease in gastric cancer. Three published series [2, 6, 8] do not include any data on lymph node status, whereas four series have addressed the use of laparoscopy in the assessment of nodal disease. Possik et al. [1] found that laparoscopy correctly identified nodal metastases in 86 of 190 patients on the basis of size alone. However, there were 71 false negatives reflecting the fact that no biopsy was performed intraoperatively and size alone is a poor predictor of involvement. Other investigators have found similar results [3, 5–7].

Bartlett et al. [27] reported a single case of gastric cancer in which LUS accurately defined N0 lymph node status preoperatively, and Finch et al. [28] showed that LUS accurately defined N stage in 89% of a series of patients with gastric cancer. LUS understaged nodal status in 11%, but no patients were overstaged with this modality.

Tio et al. [24] examined the accuracy of EUS in staging lymph nodes in 76 patients with cancer of the stomach. Lymph node metastases were correctly diagnosed in 43 of 50 patients, with a false negative diagnosis in 7 patients. No false positive diagnoses were made; however, correct staging, according to the separate definitions of N1 and N2 disease, was made in only 39 patients.

Ziegler et al. [26] compared CT scan and EUS in the diagnosis of lymph nodes involved by tumor using a CT definition of involvement as a diameter of 8 mm or greater. Of the 44 cases with histologically positive lymph nodes CT scan understaged 20 patients as N0. CT correctly predicted nodal metastases in either the N1 or N2 levels in 29 of 50 tumors. In comparison, EUS correctly identified 36 of 58 patients with involved lymph nodes, with 18 false negative examinations and 4 patients as N1 instead of N2.

M Stage (category)

Hepatic Metastases

Stell et al. [7] demonstrated that laparoscopy was significantly better at detecting hepatic metastases than transabdominal US or CT scan. Of 27 hepatic metastases in 65 patients with gastric cancer, 26 were correctly identified with laparoscopy compared with 10 by US and 14 by CT scan. The lesion missed on laparoscopy was small and lay posteriorly. Davies et al. [17] showed that spiral CT correctly detected four of seven liver metastases but also missed three (2 were small:

<10 mm) subcapsular lesions. In comparison Tio et al. [24] used EUS to correctly demonstrate hepatic metastases in one of four patients, with the remaining three patients not being assessed because of the limited penetration depth of EUS.

Possik et al. [1] found that laparoscopy correctly identified 41 of 258 patients with liver metastases and 208 without liver disease. There were three false positives where benign liver lesions were interpreted as metastatic disease without the benefit of a biopsy, emphasizing the importance of intraoperative frozen section analysis. In addition, there were six false negatives in patients with adhesions or metastases located high in segments 7 and 8, where direct visualization with the laparoscope is difficult. Other investigators have found laparoscopy to have a sensitivity of 90%–100% and specificity of up to 100% [2–8] for the detection of hepatic disease. The addition of LUS may increase the accuracy of laparoscopy in locating hepatic lesions, although Finch et al. [28] found that the majority of liver metastases can be visualized directly and that LUS detected only one liver metastasis not seen via the laparoscope in a series of 26 patients with gastric cancer. LUS can be helpful to adjudicate equivocal lesions seen on CT scan, especially small cysts or hemangiomas.

Peritoneal Metastases

Traditionally peritoneal metastases, characteristic of the biology of gastric cancer, have been the most problematic for the surgeon to diagnose. Often a few millimeters in size and widely distributed throughout the parietal and visceral peritoneum, they are often impossible to visualize with either CT scan or transabdominal US, although their presence may be inferred from ascites.

Stell et al. [7] compared laparoscopy, transabdominal US, and CT scan in the detection of peritoneal metastases. Of 13 cases with peritoneal disease, 9 were detected by laparoscopy, 3 by US, and 1 by CT scan. All patients identified by US had ascites, and the presence of metastatic disease was inferred from this. Of the four false negatives reported by laparoscopy all were presented in areas traditionally difficult to access with the laparoscope (transverse mesocolon, posterior surface of the greater omentum, diaphragm, and anterior surface of the pancreas). Peritoneal metastases were diagnosed in one of two patients with EUS [24]. In comparison, Davies et al. [17] showed that spiral CT identified 12 of 17 cases of peritoneal metastases, although there were 6 false positive examinations.

Possik et al. [1] reported a nearly 5% false positive rate from laparoscopy without the use of confirmatory frozen section analysis of suspicious peritoneal nodules, emphasizing the importance of pathological confirmation of peritoneal abnormalities. Most investigators report an average 5% false negative rate due to the presence of intra-abdominal adhesions preventing thorough abdominal examination [3, 4–8] or the presence of peritoneal disease in difficult-to-access sites such as the transverse mesocolon [3, 8] or in the lesser sac [6]. Thus a clear laparoscopic examination should not prevent the performance of a laparotomy once the decision to proceed to open operation has been made.

Table 1. The accuracy of available staging modalities for TNM staging of distal esophageal and gastroesophageal junction cancers (accuracy=number of correct examinations/total number of examinations)

	T stage [reference]	N stage [reference]	Peritoneal metastases [reference]	Hepatic metastases [reference]
Laparoscopy	–	96% [9]	96% [9]	98% [4, 9]
Endoscopic ultrasound	90% [9]	85% [24]	50% [24]	25% [24]
Transabdominal ultrasound	–	82% [9]	88% [9]	98% [4, 9]
CT scan	50% [17]	90% [9]	88% [9]	96% [4, 9, 13]

Peritoneal Cytology

The role of peritoneal lavage cytology was assessed by Burke et al. [15], who looked at those patients who returned positive lavage cytology in the absence of macroscopic peritoneal disease. Significantly, these investigators found that the prognosis of these patients was identical to that of patients with stage IV disease. This indicates that positive lavage cytology indicates microscopic peritoneal metastatic disease. These patients behave in a manner identical to patients with macroscopic peritoneal or hepatic metastases, and they should therefore be staged as M1.

Optimal Staging Technique in Gastric Cancer

The accuracies of the available staging modalities for distal esophageal and gastroesophageal junction tumors are presented in Table 1. The most accurate method of T staging is EUS, which will correctly stage the primary tumor in 90% of examinations. Failures with this technique occur when inflammation after radiation therapy or biopsy or in ulcerated lesions distorts the anatomy of the esophageal wall, whereas in more advanced lesions luminal stenosis preventing passage of the endoscope may limit the value of the examination. Laparoscopy is useful in assessing para-aortic and celiac axis lymph nodes and serves as a useful addition to EUS, which is most accurate in assessing paraesophageal nodes. For the assessment of metastatic disease to both the peritoneum and the liver, laparoscopy is the procedure of choice but is complemented by spiral CT scanning, which is effective in defining intrahepatic lesions but overlooks small peripheral or subcapsular deposits. In comparison, laparoscopy may overlook intrahepatic disease and deposits lying in segments 7 and 8.

The accuracy of the available staging modalities for gastric body carcinoma is presented in Table 2. For T stage, laparoscopy and EUS achieve comparable results, and LUS does not appear to add much to the assessment of T stage over and

Table 2. The accuracy of available staging modalities for TNM staging of distal stomach cancers (accuracy=number of correct examinations/total number of examinations)

	T stage [reference]	N stage [reference]	Peritoneal metastases [reference]	Hepatic metastases [reference]
Laparoscopy	81% [1, 5]	58% [1, 5]	94% [1, 3, 4, 8]	96% [1, 6, 8]
Laparoscopic ultrasound	82% [28]	89% [28]	–	98% [28, 29]
Endoscopic ultrasound	83% [26]	66% [26]	–	25% [26]
Transabdominal ultrasound	–	–	23% [7]	37% [7]
CT scan	66% [17]	62% [26]	71% [7, 17]	95% [7, 17]

above what can be deduced from mobility of the primary lesion and the findings of macroscopic serosal penetration. LUS is the procedure of choice for the assessment of lymph node status in that it permits the definition of abnormal nodes not only on size criteria but also on echotexture. Laparoscopy and LUS are also the most accurate methods to define both peritoneal and hepatic metastases supplemented by spiral CT scan to assess the liver parenchyma and segments 7 and 8.

The Effect of Laparoscopic Staging on Tumor Management

The management algorithm for gastric and gastroesophageal malignancy at Memorial Sloan-Kettering Cancer Center is presented in Fig. 1. All patients with biopsy-proven lesions of the distal esophagus, gastroesophageal junction, and stomach are assessed with upper gastrointestinal endoscopy, possibly with EUS, and a spiral CT of the chest, abdomen, and pelvis. All patients are then laparoscoped to determine M status and/or the risk of recurrence (T/N stage). Patients with T1N0 and T2N0 disease are managed with surgical resection. Patients with T3/T4 or T2/3 and N1 disease are considered for preoperative neoadjuvant chemotherapy and later surgical resection. Patients with metastatic disease (M1) are offered enrollment in trials of investigational chemotherapy, and then patients initially managed with chemotherapy who show good treatment response may be restaged with a view to resection.

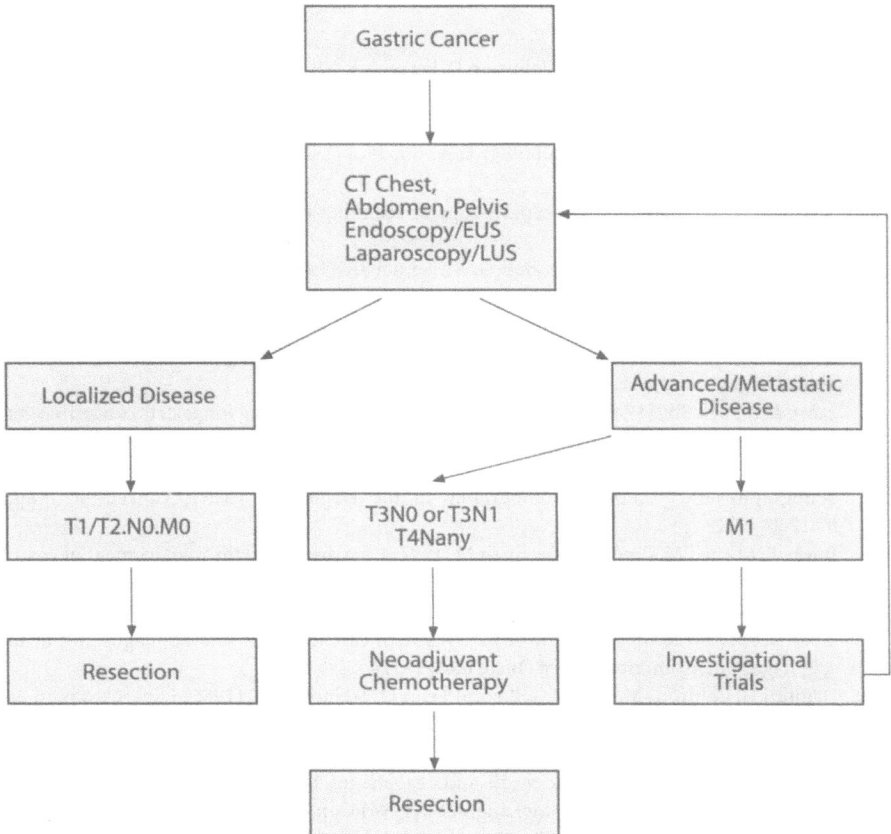

Fig. 1. Management algorithm for gastric cancer

Conclusions

In the last 5 years the management of gastric carcinoma has evolved from being primarily based on either palliative or curative surgical resection to a more complex plan incorporating neoadjuvant chemotherapy and, in the case of distal esophageal lesions, radiation therapy as well. Laparoscopic staging of patients with these carcinomas has enabled the surgeon to accurately define patients with localized lesions suitable for immediate resection and to accurately stage patients with advanced or metastatic disease more suitable for neoadjuvant therapy while sparing them the morbidity of a laparotomy. Because survival after resections for advanced gastric cancer has not changed in the last 60 years despite great advances in surgical technique, multimodality therapy aided by laparoscopy may represent a significant step forward in the rational and humane management of this disease.

References

1. Possik R, Franco E, Delmas P, Wohnrath D, Ferreira E (1986) Sensitivity, specificity and predictive value of laparoscopy for the staging of gastric cancer and for the detection of liver metastases. Cancer 58:1–6
2. Gross E, Bancewicz J, Ingram G (1984) Assessment of gastric cancer by laparoscopy. Br Med J 288:1577
3. Shandall A, Johnson C (1985) Laparoscopy or scanning in oesophageal and gastric cancer. Br J Surg 72:449–451
4. Watt I, Stewart I, Anderson D, Bell G, Anderson JR (1989) Laparoscopy, ultrasound and computed tomography in cancer of the oseophagus and gastric cardia: a prospective comparison for detecting intra-abdominal metastases. Br J Surg 76:1036–1039
5. Kriplani A, Kapur B (1991) Laparoscopy for pre-operative staging and assessment of operability in gastric cancer. Gastrointest Endos 37:441–443
6. Lowy A, Mansfield P, Leach S, Ajani J (1996) Laparoscopic staging for gastric cancer. Surgery 119:611–614
7. Stell D, Carter C, Stewart I, Anderson J (1996) Prospective comparison of laparoscopy, ultrasonography and computed tomography in the staging of gastric cancer. Br J Surg 83:1260–1262
8. Burke E, Karpeh M, Conlon K, Brennan M (1997) Laparoscopy in the management of gastric adenocarcinoma. Ann Surg 225:262–267
9. Bonavina L, Incarbone R, Lattuada E, Segalin A, Cesana B, Peracchia A (1997) Preoperative laparoscopy in the management of patients with carcinoma of the esophagus and of the esophagogastric junction. J Surg Oncol 65:171–174
10. Dagnini G, Caldroni M, Marin G, Buzzaccarini O, Tremolada C (1986) Laparoscopy in abdominal staging of esophageal carcinoma. Gastrointest Endosc 32:400–402
11. Malloy RG, McCourtney JS, Anderson JR (1995) Laparoscopy in the management of patients with cancer of the gastric cardia and oesophagus. Br J Surg 82:352–354
12. Krasna MJ, Flowers JL, Attar S, McLaughlin J (1996) Combined thoracoscopic/laparoscopic staging of esophageal cancer. J Thorac Cardiovasc Surg 111:800–807
13. O'Brien MG, Fitzgerald EF, Lee G, Crowley M, Shanahan F, O'Sullivan GC (1995) A prospective comparison of laparoscopy and imaging in staging of esophagogastric cancer before surgery. Am J Gastroenterology 90:2191–2194
14. Karpeh MS, Burke EC, Conlon KC, Brennan MF (1997) Laparoscopy: no longer optional in the evaluation of advanced gastric cancer. In: Siewert JR, Ruder JD (eds) Progress in Gastric Cancer Research. Monduzzi Editore S.p.A, Bologna, Italy, pp 131–135
15. Burke EC, Karpeh MS, Conlon KC, Brennan MF (1998) Peritoneal lavage cytology in gastric cancer: An independent predictor of outcome. Ann Surg Oncology 5:411–415
16. D'Urgo DU, Coppola R, Persiani R, Ranconi P, Caracciolo F, Picciocchi A (1996) Immediately preoperative laparoscopic staging for gastric cancer. Surg Endosc 10:996–999
17. Davies J, Chalmers AG, Sue-Ling HM, May J, Miller GV, Martin IG, Johnston D (1997) Spiral computed tomography and operative staging of gastric carcinoma: a comparison with histopathological staging. Gut 41:314–319
18. Viste A, Haugstvedt T, Eide E, Soreide O (1988) Postoperative complications and mortality after surgery for gastric cancer. Ann Surg 207:7–13
19. Hallissey M, Allum W, Roginski C, Fielding J (1988) Palliative surgery for gastric cancer. Cancer 62:440–444
20. Valen B, Viste A, Haugstvedt T, Eide E, Soreide O (1988) Treatment of gastric cancer, a national experience. Br J Surg 75:708–712

21. Kelsen D (1996) Adjuvant and neoadjuvant therapy for gastric cancer. Sem Oncol 23:379–389
22. Jarnagin WR, Bodniewicz J, Dougherty E, Conlon K, Blumgart LH, Fong Y (2000) A secondary prospective analysis of staging laparoscopy in patients with primary and secondary hepatobiliary malignancies. J Gastrointestinal Surg 4:24–43
23. American Joint Committee on Cancer (1997) AJCC Cancer Staging Manual. Lippincott-Raven Publishers, New York
24. Tio TL, Coene PP, Schouwink MH, Tytgat GN (1989) Esophagogastric carcinoma: Preoperative TNM classification with endosonography. Radiology 173:411–417
25. Ziegler K, Sanft C, Friedrich M, Stein H, Riecken EO (1991) Evaluation of endosonography in TN staging of esophageal cancer. Gut 32:16–20
26. Ziegler K, Sanft C, Zimmer T, Felsenberg D, Stein H, Deutschmann C, Riecken EO (1993) Comparison of computed tomography, endosonography, and intraoperative assessment in TN staging of gastric carcinoma. Gut 34:602–610
27. Bartlett D, Conlon K, Gerdes H, Karpeh M (1995) Laparoscopic ultrasonography: The best pretreatment staging modality in gastric adenocarcinoma? Case report. Surgery 118:562–566
28. Finch M, John T, Garden O, Allan P, Paterson-Brown S (1997) Laparoscopic ultrasonography for staging gastroesophageal cancer. Surgery 121:10–17
29. Stein HJ, Kraemer SJ, Feussner H, Fink U, Siewert JR (1997) Clinical value of diagnostic laparoscopy with laparoscopic ultrasound in patients with cancer of the esophagus or cardia. J Gastrointestinal Surg 1:167–173

Extended Diagnostic Laparoscopy in Gastric Cancer

H. Feussner · S.J.M. Kraemer · J.R. Siewert

Introduction

Imaging of abdominal organs has greatly improved with the introduction of ultrasonography (US), computed tomography (CT), and magnetic resonance imaging (MRI). Nevertheless, major discrepancies between preoperative and perioperative tumor staging in gastric cancer still occur. Accurate detection of intra-abdominal metastasis and reliable definition of local spread of the primary tumor are of considerable importance in surgical oncology [2, 3, 22].

Diagnostic laparoscopy has become well established as an important tool to improve decision making in abdominal surgery [1, 10, 17, 18, 19]. The so-called extended diagnostic laparoscopy (EDL) is used as part of the preoperative staging diagnosis. Laparoscopic ultrasound (LUS) [20, 23, 24] and intraoperative diagnostic lavage for detection of free tumor cells in the abdominal cavity [21] are obligatory parts of the EDL. This technique has the ability to extend and improve diagnostic precision in patients with abdominal tumors and in patients with pathological findings of unknown identity. Currently, we perform EDL in addition to the imaging methods mentioned above.

The objectives for the use of EDL in gastric cancer are to determine the T stage of gastric tumors with greater precision than established imaging methods can provide. Endoscopic ultrasound today provides the highest precision for preoperative estimation of T and N stages [5, 7]. However, its meaningfulness is limited by the range of the scanner and its means of application. Images can only be obtained in a range of up to 2–3 cm beyond the lumen in which the endoscope is placed and along the reach or the length of the endoscope. Therefore, the greatest part of the abdomen cannot be reached directly by endoscopic ultrasound.

Consequently, the staging of gastric cancer is usually completed by percutaneous ultrasound examination and/or CT scan to identify distant metastases, involvement of distant lymph nodes, and peritoneal spread.

The diagnostic accuracy of both of these methods is not as high as required.

Indication for EDL in Gastric Cancer

The inclusion criteria are T3 or T4 or N+ gastric carcinoma according to endoluminal ultrasound. The exclusion criteria include those patients with suspected extended adhesions after prior surgeries and those with heart and lung insufficiency or other severe heart or lung conditions.

▌ Technique

Surgeon, assistant, and scrub nurse are placed as depicted (Fig. 1). If one monitor is used, it is preferably placed above the head of the patient.

After the pneumoperitoneum has been established, the EDL begins with the introduction of an 11-mm trocar at the umbilicus (Fig. 2). A 30° 10-mm laparoscope is then introduced into the abdominal cavity. The 30° optic allows inspection of areas such as the right subphrenic space or the Douglas space in the pelvis.

When the laparoscope has been inserted, the second trocar is then placed under visual control between the lower and upper quadrant as shown. Through this trocar a retractor may be introduced to lift up the liver or other organs. Before any further manipulations the diagnostic laparoscopy begins with the inspection of the upper abdominal cavity. The patient is brought into a 30°–45° anti-Trendelenburg position. This brings the omentum and the small and large intestine caudad, exposing the organs of the upper abdomen.

As mentioned above, the laparoscopic procedure is always performed in the same order (Fig. 3), beginning with the left upper abdomen and continuing counterclockwise to the right upper abdomen and the right lower abdomen. From here, one turns clockwise to the left lower quadrant, giving the omentum and the small bowel a closer look.

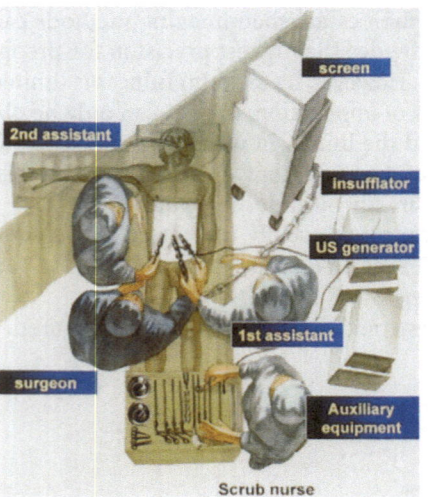

Fig. 1. Positioning of the patient, the surgical team, and the video turret

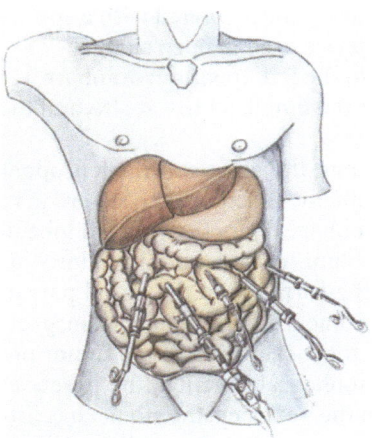

Fig. 2. Trocar placement

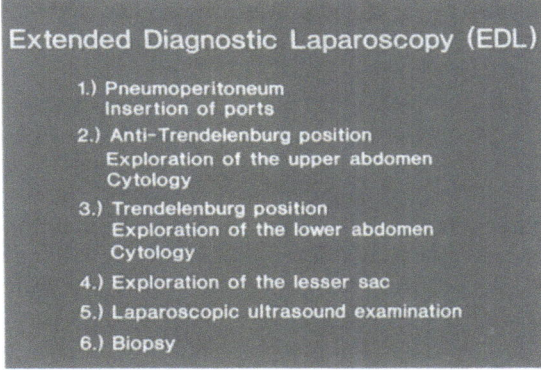

Fig. 3. Standardized protocol for the EDL procedure

Extended Diagnostic Laparoscopy (EDL)

1.) Pneumoperitoneum
    Insertion of ports
2.) Anti-Trendelenburg position
    Exploration of the upper abdomen
    Cytology
3.) Trendelenburg position
    Exploration of the lower abdomen
    Cytology
4.) Exploration of the lesser sac
5.) Laparoscopic ultrasound examination
6.) Biopsy

The first inspection ends with the examination of the lower left quadrant and the organs of the pelvic space. Thus the laparoscopic exploration follows roughly the pattern of an „S".

The inspection is carried out to find pathological changes in the serosa and the visceral and parietal peritoneum, adhesions that may be caused by tumor spread, and bulges or lumps caused by lymph nodes or tumor masses. Local tumor spread and small superficially located metastases of liver and spleen can be visualized with this method, as well as small lymph node metastasis in the omentum and smaller amounts of ascites that to date cannot be detected with the very advanced imaging methods available. Such findings may prompt a dramatic change in the treatment course if a multimodal approach to the treatment of gastric cancer (and other tumors) is applied.

After the initial overview and before any further manipulations, diagnostic lavage is performed to detect free tumor cells. Physiological saline solution

(200 ml) is instilled into the upper abdominal cavity and aspirated with a special suction device similar to the standard suction device used in open surgery.

Two additional ports are then introduced into the left upper quadrant. An 11-mm trocar is inserted cephalad and lateral from the umbilical trocar site, and the next trocar is placed just lateral from this port.

After the first overview, the abdominal wall and the organs of the left upper abdominal cavity are carefully inspected individually. To expose the lesser curve of the stomach and the hiatus with the gastroesophageal junction, the left lobe of the liver must be elevated with a retractor or a blunt instrument. This allows inspection of the anterior aspect of the fundus, the corpus, and the antral part of the stomach. The lesser sac and the area of the celiac trunk can easily be inspected after dividing the gastrohepatic ligament. If the localization of the tumor necessitates a closer investigation of the gastroesophageal junction, the phrenoesophageal ligament may be partially divided. In the next step, the stomach is lifted up close to the greater curve left of the pylorus with a Babcock or Allison clamp to elevate and stretch the greater omentum. This is then divided, opening a window in the greater omentum that allows direct inspection of the retrogastric space and posterior wall of the stomach (Fig. 4). The anterior aspect of the corpus and the head of the pancreas can also be inspected as well as the celiac axis.

The spleen is examined next. By carefully pulling the left edge of the greater omentum caudally, the spleen can be visualized.

The anterior and posterior aspects of the left lobe of the liver can be examined by lifting it up with a retractor. The consistency of the liver can be tested with a blunt instrument, which can also provide the first hints of liver metastasis deep within the liver parenchyma. By moving the laparoscope to the right upper abdomen the right lobe of the liver can be examined. The right subphrenic and the anterior aspect of the liver can be seen easily. With a fan retractor or a similar device the liver can be elevated and the posterior aspect partially inspected by simply turning the laparoscope axially 180°. Inspection of the gallbladder, common duct and round ligament, pylorus and duodenum can be easily achieved.

Now the patient is brought into a 30° Trendelenburg position. This brings the gut into the upper half of the abdominal cavity, thus exposing the pelvic organs. The abdominal wall, ileocecal junction, colon, sigmoid, and rectum can be given a closer look. The mesentery can be checked for peritoneal carcinosis.

Because peritoneal secondary metastasis to the ovaries (Krukenberg tumors) play a great role in the prognosis in gastric cancer in women, the pelvic organs must be inspected very carefully. This can be achieved easily with blunt forceps. A small amount of ascites is frequently found, especially in women, and suctioned for cytological investigation.

After the inspection of the lower half of the abdomen, the patient is brought back into the 30° anti-Trendelenburg position. The laparoscope is moved to the left 11-mm trocar and a special 10-mm flexible LUS probe is inserted into the umbilical port (Fig. 5). To avoid artifacts, LUS should be performed before any biopsies are taken. The LUS procedure is videotaped as well, using a screen divider so that the laparoscopic view and the ultrasound image can be seen on the same screen at the same time. In this fashion, the organs of the upper quadrants can be easily examined with LUS. The flexible head of the ultrasound probe fol-

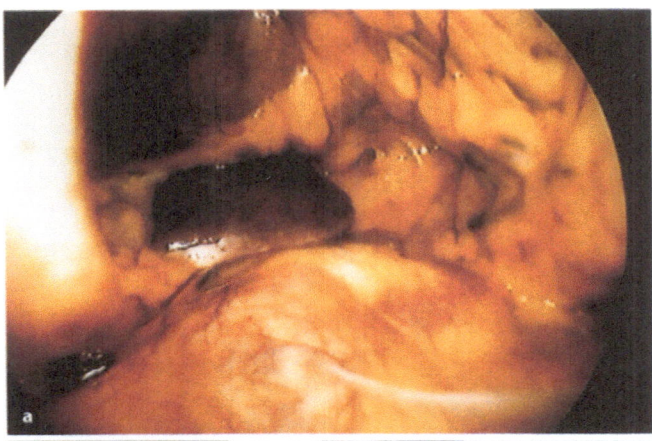

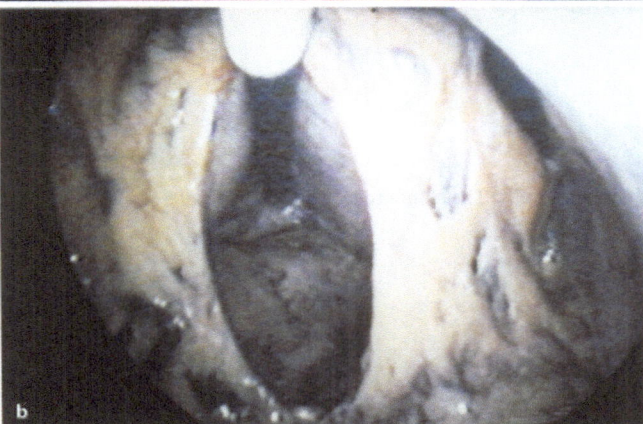

Fig. 4a, b. Exploration of the retrogastric space (lesser sac): A window through the gastrocolic ligament permits access to the posterior gastric wall, the pancreas, and the hilus of the spleen

lows the surface of the liver without problem, guaranteeing good contact with the surface and high resolution. This method allows the detection of small liver metastases (≤1 cm) or the differentiation between liver metastases, cysts, and hemangioma. To judge the T stage of gastric carcinoma, the stomach is filled with 250–300 ml of saline (hydrosonography) by the anesthesiologist via the nasogastric tube, which we always have in place during any laparoscopic procedure. If necessary, an equal amount of saline may be instilled into the upper abdomen to further improve the quality of the LUS image. This trick allows checking for tumor invasion of gastric cancer into the pancreas or for enlarged lymph nodes. Especially in thin patients, tumor invasion from gastric cancer into adjacent organs is almost undetectable for the radiologist because in these patients there is no layer of fatty tissue between the organs.

By moving the LUS probe from the umbilical port into a third port, which may be introduced in the right upper quadrant, the stomach and the adjacent organs can be investigated thoroughly, and any spot of the abdominal cavity may be reached with the LUS probe.

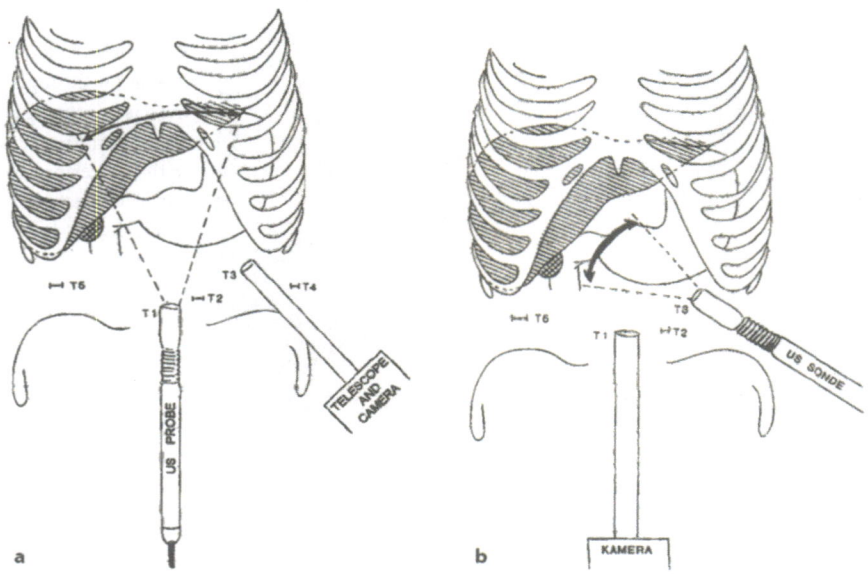

Fig. 5a, b. Laparoscopic ultrasonography: The standard evaluation is completed by a lateral transection

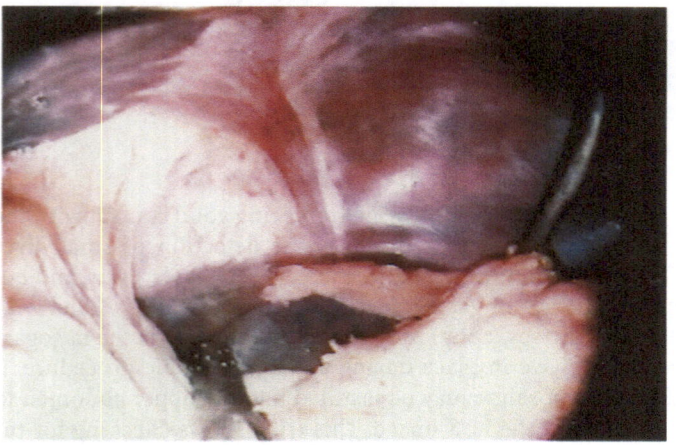

Fig. 6. A special 10-mm suction device is introduced to perform the abdominal lavage for free tumor cells

After biopsies have been taken, another diagnostic lavage is performed as described above. This lavage serves as a control of whether tumor cells have been spread during the surgical manipulations. To kill off potentially free tumor cells we routinely rinse the abdomen at the end of EDL with taurolidine (Fig. 6).

Practical Aspects of EDL

Because of the growing experience with laparoscopic operations, extended diagnostic laparoscopy can today be performed in principle in all cases. If patients who are not fit for an operation at all (and in whom the laparoscopic exploration would not be indicated) are excluded, only those patients in whom previous major abdominal surgery has been performed may present difficulties.

In our own controlled series of 111 patients, laparoscopy could not be completed for technical reasons in 4 patients (3,6%); 3 patients were found to have dense intra-abdominal adhesions of unknown origin; and in 1 patient the investigation could not be performed because of equipment failure.

The median investigation time ranges between 30 and 60 min [own results: 47 min (range: 23–111 min)]. The morbidity and mortality rates of EDL are low.

Diagnostic Yield of EDL

A considerable number of studies are available to analyze the objective amount of information that can be obtained by diagnostic laparoscopy in gastric cancer and the relative gain in information compared with other modern imaging procedures.

Surgical laparoscopy of today has to compete with helical CT, a new generation of transcutaneous ultrasound, endoluminal ultrasound, and MRI. Therefore, we will focus in this chapter on the more recent studies on extended diagnostic laparoscopy and sophisticated methods of imaging procedures.

The respective importance of the different diagnostic options should be delineated according to the TNM classification.

Modification of the Tumor Stage by Laparoscopy

In 56 of 111 patients (50.5%) the findings at laparoscopy were identical to those of prelaparoscopic imaging methods. In 6 of 111 patients (5.4%), laparoscopy revealed additional findings besides the gastric tumor important enough to alter the treatment management. Five patients were found to have liver cirrhosis as confirmed by biopsy. In one patient, a previously unknown ovarian carcinoma was detected.

In 17 of 111 patients (15.3%) the tumor was downgraded through laparoscopy and biopsy. Tumor invasion of the liver was suspected before EDL, in 6 of 111 (5.4%) patients there was invasion of the pancreas, invasion of the diaphragm in 2 of 111 (1.8%), and peritoneal spread in 4 of 111 (3.6%).

The tumor was upstaged in 28 of 111 patients (25.2%). Peritoneal secondaries were found in 26 of 111 (23%) patients, infiltration of adjacent organs in 3 of 111 (2.7%), and distant metastases in 4of 111 (3.6%; 3 hepatic, 1 colonic). Overall, detailed laparoscopy plus laparoscopic ultrasound altered the preoperative diagnosis in 51 of 111 patients (46.0%), with advanced gastric cancer leading to changes in management in 45 of 111 (40.5%) patients.

In those patients in whom laparoscopy showed a lower tumor stage, infiltration of adjacent organs was excluded (18 patients). This resulted in a change from T4 to T2 classification in nine patients. All underwent primary resection according to our protocol. The findings at operation and the result of the pathological report confirmed the results of laparoscopy. Four patients in whom peritoneal spread could be excluded by laparoscopy were treated by preoperative chemotherapy. Chemotherapy could be avoided in 26 patients found to have peritoneal secondaries.

Overall, the planned management had to be changed in 45 of 51 patients in whom the diagnosis was altered by laparoscopy (including the 6 patients with additional laparoscopic findings) or 40.5% of the group of 111 patients.

Inspection of the Lesser Sac

The diagnostic importance of the separate inspection of the lesser sac was analyzed in detail. An adequate staging of the tumor would not have been possible in 11 patients unless the lesser sac was entered. In the majority of cases, this was due to peritoneal spread or pancreatic infiltration (Table 1).

Laparoscopic Ultrasound

LUS gave decisive additional information in eight cases. In three instances this led to an upstaging, whereas in five cases a downstaging could be achieved (7.2% of the whole group or 15.7% of these in whom the diagnosis had to be changed).

Detection of Liver Metastases

According to the inclusion criteria, no patient had known liver or other metastases as the result of the clinical staging including the different imaging techniques. Laparoscopy and LUS, however, revealed three cases of liver metastases. In another patient, a large metastasis in the transverse colon (Table 2) was detected.

Assessment of Peritoneal Spread

In six cases, peritoneal spread was suspected but not proven prelaparoscopically (4 because of ascites as seen during EUS and CT scan and 2 because of a diffuse thickening of the omentum on CT). The presence of peritoneal carcinomatosis was confirmed by laparoscopy in two cases. In another four patients, it could be ruled out both by the macroscopic aspect as well as by cytology. On the other hand, peritoneal secondaries were found in as many as 26 patients in whom they were not suspected before EDL (Table 3).

Infliction of Adjacent Organs

Invasion of neighboring organs was suspected in 26 cases in clinical staging. This could be confirmed by laparoscopy in 8 instances but ruled out in as many as 18 cases. On the other hand, three additional cases previously unsuspected of tumor invasion were found (Table 4).

Table 1. Diagnostic yield of the preparation of the lesser sac

Preparation of the lesser sac successful	$n=107/111$
No additional information	$n=96$
Decisive additional information	$n=11$
Infiltration of the pancreas	$n=4$
Peritoneal spread	$n=44$
No infiltration of the gastric serosa (=T2)	$n=3$

Table 2. Detection of liver metastases

Prelaparoscopic staging	Laparoscopy	Laparoscopy + LUS
$n=0/111$	$n=1/111$	$n=3/111$

Table 3. Assessment of peritoneal spread

Prelaparoscopic staging	Laparoscopy + cytology
Peritoneal spread suspected	$n=6$
Peritoneal spread confirmed	$n=2$
Ruled out	$n=4$
Not suspected	$n=105$
Absence of p.c. confirmed	$n=79$
Proven	$n=26$

Table 4. Infliction of adjacent organs

Prelaparoscopic staging	Laparoscopy + LUS
No invasion	$n=85$
Confirmed	$n=82$
Invasion confirmed (T4)	$n=3$
T4	$n=26$
Confirmed	$n=8$
No invasion (T3)	$n=18$

Comparison of Prelaparoscopic and Laparoscopic Staging with Intraoperative Findings

In contrast to the primary intention, laparotomy was performed in 44 patients within 72 h after laparoscopy. This subgroup included nine patients who had been found to belong to the T2 stage and thus were suitable for primary gastric resection without previous chemotherapy. In all of them, a R0 resection could be achieved.

In another six patients, chemotherapy was refused or not performed despite the original intention. Nine patients were operated on for palliative reasons. Laparoscopic staging was correct in 42 of 44 cases (95,4%).

In one of the false negative patients, chemotherapy had originally been considered but later on was refused by the patient. During total gastrectomy, cholecystectomy was also performed because of concurrent cholecystolithiasis. Histopathological examination revealed a tiny spot of peritoneal carcinomatosis on the gallbladder that had not been detected macroscopically.

In another patient who underwent subtotal gastrectomy for palliation of malignant gastric outlet syndrome with known peritoneal spread, an additional liver metastasis was found.

▌ Discussion

At present we define three main treatment options for gastric cancer. The first option is primary resection in patients with a localized lesion. The second option is preoperative chemotherapy in the attempt to downstage subjects with advanced disease. The third treatment option is symptomatic or palliative treatment only for those patients with disseminated disease. It is known that the results of nonradical surgery are disappointing [8]. Similarly in advanced disease it is recognized that chemotherapy has little to offer.

Accurate preoperative evaluation of patients with gastric cancer is therefore indispensable to the treatment of the disease. If a tumor is overstaged, this could lead to an overly aggressive strategy of treatment or, even worse, to therapeutic resignation. If it is understaged, a higher rate of nonradical resections or nonresective laparotomies must be accepted. Accordingly, modern management of patients with cancer seeks to accurately stage and plan treatment before embarking on any form of therapy. Conventional open diagnostic laparotomy is the most reliable method for ascertaining tumor stage in patients with gastric cancer. Because of the morbidity and mortality of this procedure, it is not routinely performed before definitive treatment [9]. Consequently, efforts are being made to develop less invasive yet accurate diagnostic techniques. Endosonography has been shown to evaluate the depth of tumor infiltration with an accuracy of 69%–92% [4, 6] but only an accuracy of 60.5% with regard to lymph nodes. The main indications for CT scanning and conventional ultrasound are to detect distant nodal and organ metastases.

An important diagnostic gap exists in the identification of peritoneal metastases. It is estimated that at least 14%–22% of patients with advanced gastric cancer have peritoneal carcinosis, the frequency increasing with the T stage of the tumor. Neither CT scanning nor conventional ultrasound or endosonography are adequate for this purpose, especially in cases where peritoneal or omental deposits are small and ascites is not yet present. In our study, the prevalence of peritoneal spread was in accordance with the literature (25.2%), but only two cases were correctly diagnosed by the prelaparoscopic staging, which clearly demonstrates that this diagnostic gap may only be filled by laparoscopy.

In contrast to our expectations before this study, laparoscopy/LUS were also helpful in determining the infiltration of adjacent organs (T3 or T4). Prelaparoscopic staging (endosonography/CT scan) demonstrated a clear tendency of overstaging that could successfully be corrected by diagnostic laparoscopy.

On the other hand, liver metastases were missed in three cases that were detected by laparoscopy and, in particular, laparoscopic sonography. Although this number of overlooked metastases is low, laparotomy could be avoided in these individual patients.

Conclusively, diagnostic laparoscopy is more accurate than all other established tests under investigation and relatively quick to perform with minimal morbidity and no mortality. Disadvantages include costs, the need for an experienced surgeon, and a delay in starting the treatment. A theoretical objection is the risk of tumor spread during laparoscopy. At present, however, there is no evidence that diagnostic laparoscopy in gastric cancer promotes tumor spread. We believe that any of these disadvantages are offset by the avoidance of unnecessary surgery or chemotherapy.

Our method of laparoscopy (extended diagnostic laparoscopy) differs from that described by other authors who have already evaluated the importance of laparoscopy in gastric cancer [10–13]. The lesser sac was carefully inspected, multiple biopsies were taken, and LUS of the tumor and adjacent organs was also performed. Although this series is small, we feel that these additional maneuvers are nevertheless highly effective, as confirmed by more recent studies in particular with regard to the use of ultrasound [14] and meticulous dissection including cytology [15, 16]. To fully inspect the tumor it is essential to enter the lesser sac, which led to important additional information in as much as 10% of our patients.

Cytology is important as well, because small tumor deposits can easily be missed. Multiple biopsies from suspicious areas are mandatory.

LUS proved useful to confirm or refute invasion or to show the presence of unsuspected liver metastases, being responsible for the change of diagnosis in 15.7% of our cases. It should always be an integral part of diagnostic laparoscopy.

The value of laparoscopy for the planning of treatment strategies within the multimodal therapy approach is convincing and in accordance with other studies. In almost one-quarter of our patients either undertreatment or overtreatment could be avoided. Preoperative chemotherapy, for example, turned out not to be necessary in nine patients who underwent primary surgery, and in four other patients laparoscopy ruled out previously suspected peritoneal carcinomatosis, which otherwise would have resulted in therapeutic resignations.

Overall, extended diagnostic laparoscopy altered our original therapeutic strategy in 40% of patients with advanced gastric cancer. We conclude that careful diagnostic laparoscopy using the methods described should be aimed at for the management of all patients with advanced gastric cancer.

References

1. Kraemer SJM, Stein H, Feussner H, Siewert JR (1966) Technique of extended diagnostic laparoscopy in the staging of cancer of the esophagus. Dis Esophag 9:228–235
2. Findlay M, Cunningham D (1993) Chemotherapy of carcinoma of the stomach. Cancer Treatment Rev 19:29–44
3. Siewert JR, Fink U (1992) Multimodale Therapiekonzepte bei Tumoren des Gastrointestinaltraktes. Chirurg 63:242–250
4. Takemoto T, Tada M, Dittler HJ, Rösch T, Siewert JR (1993) Impact of staging on treatment of gastric carcinoma. Endoscopy 25:46–50
5. Natterman Ch, Dancygier H (1992) Endosonographie bei Magentumoren Leber Magen Darm 6/92:211–219
6. Halpert RD, Feczko PF (1993) Role of radiology in the diagnosis and staging of gastric malignancy. Endoscopy 25:36–45
7. Rösch T, Classen M (1992) Gastroenterologie Endosonography. Thieme, Stuttgart
8. Lauren P (1965) The two histological maintypes of gastric carcinoma: Diffuse and so-called intestinal type carcinoma. Acta Pathol Microbiol Scand 64:31–43
9. Fink U, Schuhmacher C, Stein HJ, Busch R, Feussner H, Dittler HJ, Helmberger A, Böttcher K, Siewert JR (1995) Preoperative chemotherapy for stage III–IV gastric carcinoma: feasibility, response and outcome after complete resection. Br J Surg 82:1248–1252
10. Dupont JB, Lee JR, Burton GR, Cohn JI (1978) Adenocarcinoma of the stomach: review of 1497 cases. Cancer 41:941–947
11. Possik RA, Franco EL, Pires DR, Wohnrath DR, Ferreira EB (1986) Sensitivity, specificity and predictive value of laparoscopy for the staging of gastric cancer and for the detection of liver metastases. Cancer 58:1–6
12. Kriplani AK, Kapur BML (1991) Laparoscopy for the pre-operative staging and assessment of operability in gastric carcinoma. Gastrointestinal Endoscopy 37:441–443
13. Easter DW, Cushieri A, Nathanson LK, Lavelle-Jones M (1992) The utility of diagnostic laparoscopy for abdominal disorders. Arch Surg 127:379
14. Raven JL (1994) Carcinoma of the stomach. In: Misiewicz JJ, Pounder RE, Venables CW (eds) Diseases of the gut and pancreas. Blackwell Scientific, Oxford, pp 335–352
15. Finch MD, Johm TG, Garden OJ, Allan PL, Paterson-Brown S (1997) Laparoscopic ultrasonography for staging gastroesophageal cancer. Surgery 1:10–17
16. Burke EC, Karpeh MS, Conlon KC, Brennan MF (1997) Laparoscopy in the management of gastric adenocarcinoma. Ann Surg 223:262–267
17. Lowy AM, Mansfield PF, Leach SD, Ajani J (1996) Laparoscopic staging for gastric cancer. Surgery 119:611–614
18. Lightdale CJ (1992) Laparoscopy for cancer staging. Endoscopy 24:682–686
19. Molloy RG, McCourtney JS, Anderson JR (1995) Laparoscopy in the management of patients with cancer of the gastric cardia and esophagus. Br J Surg 82:352–354
20. Popova TN, Kohersky FP, Alexandrova MI (1987) Application of laparoscopy in stomach cancer staging. Vopr Oncol 33:75–78

21. Warshaw AL (1991) Implications of peritoneal cytology for staging of early pancreatic cancer. Am J Surg 1261:26–29
22. Kraemer SJM, Feussner H, Fink U, Siewert JR (1995) Erfahrungen mit der erweiterten diagnostischen Laparoskopie mit laparoskopischem Ultraschall im präoperativen Verfahren. Staging gastrointestinaler Tumoren In: Schyra B (ed) Beiträge zur klinischen Chirurgie. Shaber, Aachen, pp 91–94
23. Feussner H, Kraemer SJM, Siewert JR (1995) Wertigkeit laparoskopischer Untersuchungstechniken bei malignen Erkrankungen. Chir Gastroenterol II:268–273
24. Feussner H, Kraemer SJM, Siewert JR (1994) Technik der laparoskopischen Ultraschalluntersuchung bei der diagnostischen Laparoskopie. Langenbecks Arch Chir 379:248

Laparoscopic Staging for Pancreatic Malignancy

N.J. Espat · K.C. Conlon

Introduction

Pancreatic cancer is an uncommon malignancy with an unfavorable prognosis that occurs predominantly in the sixth and seventh decades of life. Adenocarcinoma is the most common histological type of this disease and will occur in more than 80% of patients with pancreatic cancer. At the time of diagnosis only 10% of patients have disease confined to the pancreas, 40% exhibit local spread, and 50% demonstrate distant disease (metastatic) spread [1, 2].

Approximately 28,000 new cases of pancreatic adenocarcinoma are reported each year in the United States. Surgical resection offers the only chance for long-term survival in these patients; however, less than 20% are operative candidates, because radiographically inapparent disease such as occult peritoneal or hepatic metastasis precludes curative resection [3–6].

Goal of Laparoscopic Staging

The principal goal of laparoscopic evaluation is to provide an accurate TNM staging (UICC) of the tumor and to guide stage-appropriate management [7, 8]. Once the diagnosis is confirmed and the patient is staged, the goal of treatment should be to render the patient free of tumor (UICC stage R0), because accurate disease staging and an R0 tumor stage after resection have been shown by multivariate analyses to have the greatest impact on prognosis [9]. Laparoscopic staging enables the selection of patients that will benefit from operation with the intent to cure as opposed to palliation (Fig. 1).

The Role of CT in the Staging of Pancreatic Malignancy

Laparoscopic staging in conjunction with preoperative computed tomography (CT) scanning has been shown to be an effective, accurate, and safe means of staging peripancreatic malignancy that has been previously validated by our group and others [5, 7, 10, 11].

Dynamic contrast-enhanced CT is the radiographic study of choice for the preoperative evaluation of patients with pancreatic cancer [3, 12]. However, de-

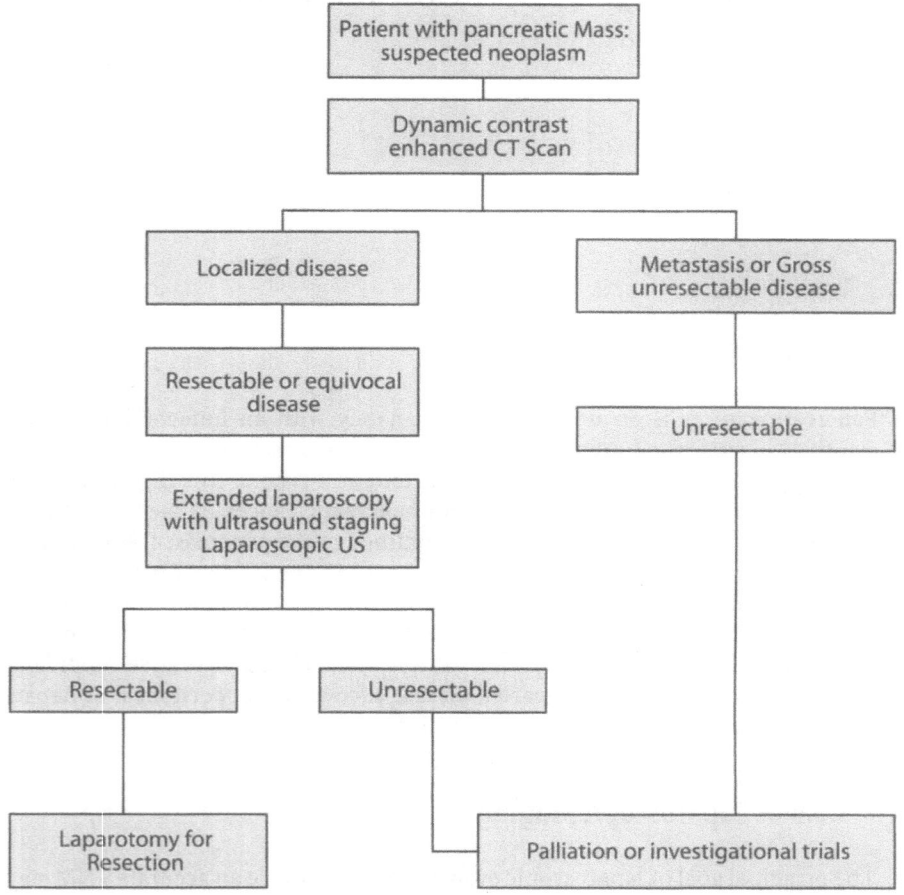

Fig. 1. Algorithm of staging procedures for pancreatic cancer

spite the advanced imaging modalities presently available to assess patients with pancreatic cancer, only a limited assessment of resectability is achieved using current CT techniques [1, 2]. Patients with unresectable pancreatic cancer have median survival of approximately 6 months, and in this patient population proceeding with a laparotomy without resection results only in significant perioperative morbidity, potential mortality, and a diminished quality of life [13, 14].

In oncological staging, the predictive accuracy of CT examination alone for resection has been a matter of controversy. CT examination alone has been compared to combined CT and laparoscopy for assessing potential resectability, with the combined approach being identified as superior [1, 2, 3, 7, 15]. Although dynamic contrast-enhanced CT has been demonstrated to be a valuable method to assess unresectability of gastrointestinal malignancy, it is less specific for the determination of resectability [1–3, 7].

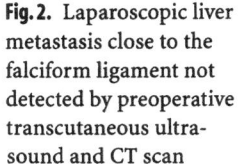

Fig.2. Laparoscopic liver metastasis close to the falciform ligament not detected by preoperative transcutaneous ultrasound and CT scan

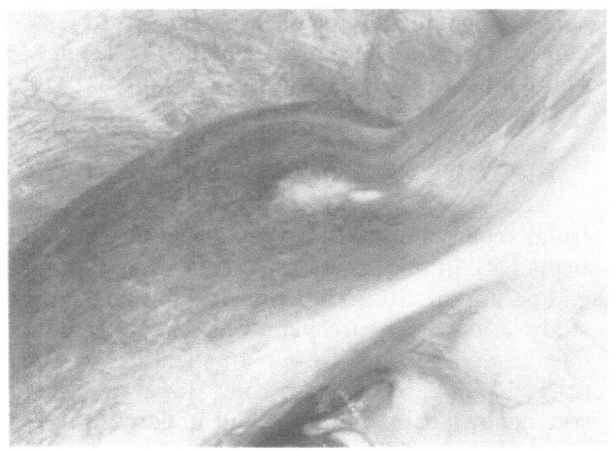

CT resolution is limited to lesions that are larger than 2–3 mm, allowing smaller lesions to be missed. CT has been demonstrated to have a high sensitivity in determining local regional extension of disease and vascular encasement, predicting unresectability in up to 100% of patients. Despite this obvious benefit, CT is far less specific at determining resectability, and reports of accurate assessment of resectability in pancreatic tumor range from 57% to 88% [3, 7, 16, 17]. In contrast, laparoscopic staging will identify subcentimeter hepatic, peritoneal, or omental tumor implants that are missed by CT examination alone (see Fig. 2) Additionally, peritoneal cytology from washings at the time of laparoscopy will identify an additional 8% of patients with micrometastases, and these have a prognosis equally poor as those with visible disease [18]. Published series report that laparoscopic staging identifies disease in 22% to 48% of patients who have no evidence of disseminated disease by CT [19–22]. As such, staging with CT alone means that many patients will still undergo a needless laparotomy without the benefit of curative resection [1, 2].

Beyond the benefit of direct organ visualization and examination for radiographically inapparent disease, laparoscopy provides access for ultrasound evaluation. In this manner, deep parenchymal metastasis and vascular involvement by tumor can be identified [8, 23].

Warshaw et al. compared several different modalities in the preoperative assessment of pancreatic cancer [15]. Dynamic CT, magnetic resonance imaging (MRI), angiography, and laparoscopy were evaluated for accuracy in this study. Of 88 patients considered to have potentially curable disease, CT was 92% accurate in determining unresectability but only 56% sensitive. Resectability was predicted in only 45% of patients. CT scanning failed to identify liver metastasis in 23 patients. Angiography predicted 25 of 26 cases as being unresectable, with a sensitivity of only 66%. The accuracy of predicting resectability was only 54%. MRI results were similar to those of CT scan and offered no advantage. Laparoscopy identified liver and peritoneal metastasis in 22 of 23 cases and was correct in not identifying metastasis in 24 of 24 patients, with an overall 98% accuracy of laparoscopy; however, of the 19 cases in which no metastasis were seen, only 8 proceeded to resection.

The Early Experience with Laparoscopy for Pancreatic Malignancy

Ishida reported in 1983 the results of limited laparoscopic examination in 71 patients [24]. In this group of patients, hepatic metastasis were identified in 30% and peritoneal disease noted in 41% of patients. In 1988 Cuschieri performed a study of immediate preoperative laparoscopy and then compared the results to open exploration [25]. Of the 51 patients, 42 were correctly staged as having unresectable disease by laparoscopy. However, of the nine patients considered resectable by laparoscopy, only four underwent resection. Warshaw, in a separate series, performed laparoscopy in 40 patients [26]. Fourteen patients had positive findings at laparoscopy that resulted in a change in their operative management. Findings at laparoscopy included hepatic metastasis in six patients, peritoneal disease in seven, and a single omental implant. In the remaining 26 patients, three additional hepatic metastases not identified by laparoscopy were identified at the time of operation.

These studies early in the modern era of laparoscopic staging highlight the predictive value of simple laparoscopy and underscore the pitfalls of a negative examination. Diagnostic laparoscopy without ultrasound or a multiport technique is reported to assess resectability in under 40% of patients. In sharp contradistinction, laparoscopic staging performed in a manner that mimics open exploration exceeds 90% accuracy at predicting resectability [7].

The Memorial Sloan-Kettering Experience

At Memorial Sloan-Kettering Cancer Center, we have instituted a multiport extended laparoscopic technique for the staging and assessment of resectability of peripancreatic tumors [7]. In our management algorithm, all patients undergo a contrast-enhanced dynamic CT scan of the abdomen for determination of obvious unresectable disease before proceeding to laparoscopy. Our laparoscopic staging technique, unlike previously published reports, mimics the surgical assessment of resectability performed at open exploration.

Management Algorithm

Patients presenting with suspected or diagnosed pancreatic cancer undergo a good-quality dynamic contrast-enhanced CT examination. As mentioned, CT scan accurately assesses unresectable disease. Unresectability by CT scan is determined if one or more of the following are present: (a) hepatic, peritoneal, or omental metastasis; (b) extrapancreatic extension of tumor (i.e., mesocolic involvement), invasion, or encasement of the celiac axis or hepatic or superior mesenteric artery [7]. Patients determined to have portal or superior mesenteric

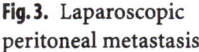
Fig. 3. Laparoscopic
peritoneal metastasis

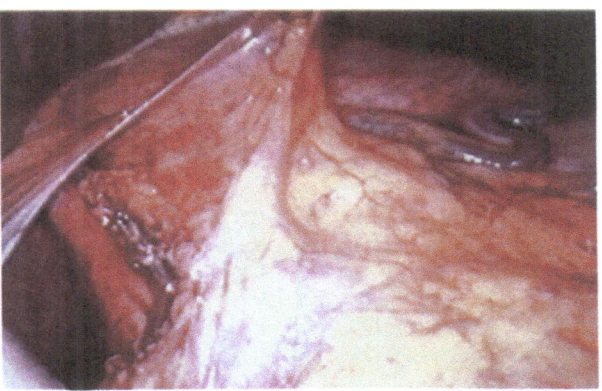

vein encroachment but not complete occlusion by tumor are considered potentially resectable and thus undergo laparoscopic staging [27].

Patients determined to have potentially resectable or equivocal disease by CT as well as those lacking histological confirmation of malignancy should then proceed to laparoscopic staging before open exploration. Findings at the time of laparoscopy will then identify a further subset of patients that are unresectable (see Fig. 3).

The Technique of Extended Laparoscopic Staging

The multiport extended laparoscopic staging we perform begins with an open technique to place a 10-mm periumbilical blunt port for the creation of a pneumoperitoneum (Fig. 4). A 30-degree angled telescope is passed through this port. Trocars are placed in the right (10 mm) and left (5 mm) upper quadrants of the abdomen. Positioning of the trochars is within the line of the planned laparotomy incision should the patient be resectable.

Initially, peritoneal inspection is performed with a systematic four-quadrant examination, searching for obvious peritoneal extension of disease. Peritoneal washings for cytological examination are collected before organ or tumor manipulation. Samples are collected after separately instilling 200 cc of saline into the right and left upper quadrants. The primary tumor is assessed, noting local extent, size, and fixation.

The patient is then placed in a 20-degree reverse Trendelenburg position with 10 degrees of left lateral tilt. Next, the anterior and posterior surfaces of the right and left lobes of the liver are visually inspected. Palpation of the liver is achieved with the use of a 10-mm instrument. The liver is retracted anteriorly, and the hepatoduodenal ligament is examined for gross adenopathy. The hilus of the liver is visualized, and the foramen of Winslow is examined. If indicated, a periportal lymph node biopsy can be performed at this time.

The patient is then repositioned into a 10-degree Trendelenburg position without tilt, and the omentum is retracted into the left upper quadrant. The liga-

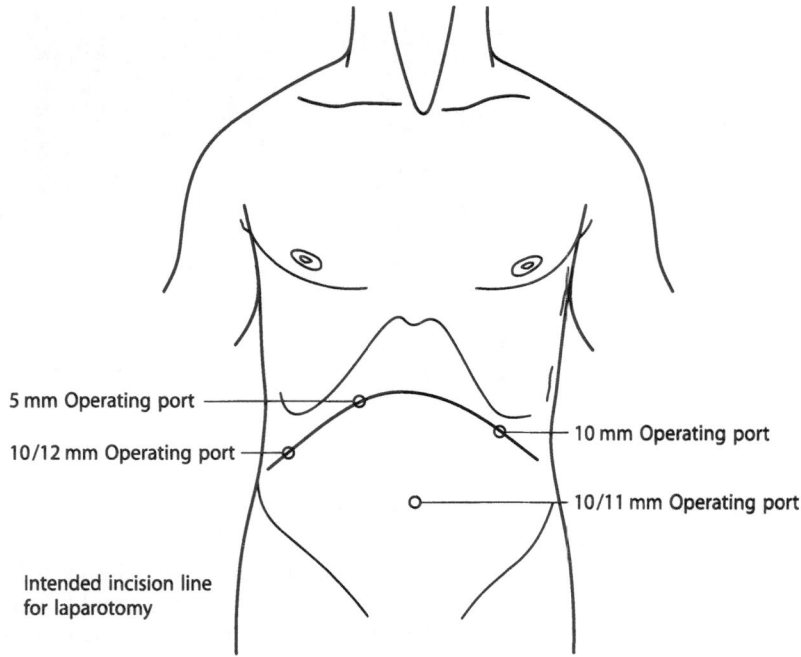

5 mm Operating port

10/12 mm Operating port

10 mm Operating port

10/11 mm Operating port

Intended incision line
for laparotomy

Fig. 4. Positioning of trocars for staging laparoscopy with respect to incision line of subsequent laparotomy

ment of Treitz is visualized, and the mesocolon is closely inspected. The patient is returned to the supine position, and the gastrohepatic omentum is incised such that the caudate lobe of the liver, vena cava, and celiac axis are exposed. Celiac, hepatic, or perigastric nodes are sampled if necessary (Fig. 5). The lesser sac is examined, and the body and tail of the pancreas are visualized (Fig. 6).

Laparoscopic ultrasound is performed on the right upper quadrant 10-mm port (Fig. 7). Evaluation for the presence of non-surface hepatic lesions is carried out in systematic fashion. Beginning at the portal vein confluence, the right and left lobes of the liver are examined. Curving the laparoscopic ultrasound probe gently toward the liver enables assessment of most of segment VIII up along the diaphragm. The pancreatic tumor is now examined by placing the ultrasound probe along the pylorus and following the duodenal sweep. Direct evaluation over the head of the pancreas is also accomplished. The relationship of the portomesenteric confluence to the superior mesenteric artery is noted (Fig. 8).

Unresectability at laparoscopy is determined if one or more of the following are confirmed histologically: (1) hepatic, serosal, peritoneal, or omental metastasis; (2) extrapancreatic extension of tumor; (3) celiac or high portal vein involvement by tumor; (4) invasion or encasement of the celiac axis, hepatic artery, or superior mesenteric artery.

If venous involvement by tumor is less than the entire retropancreatic portal vein, then the patient is considered potentially resectable and will undergo exploration for potential pancreaticoduodenectomy.

Fig. 5. Laparoscopic perigastric lymph node and excitional lymph node biopsy

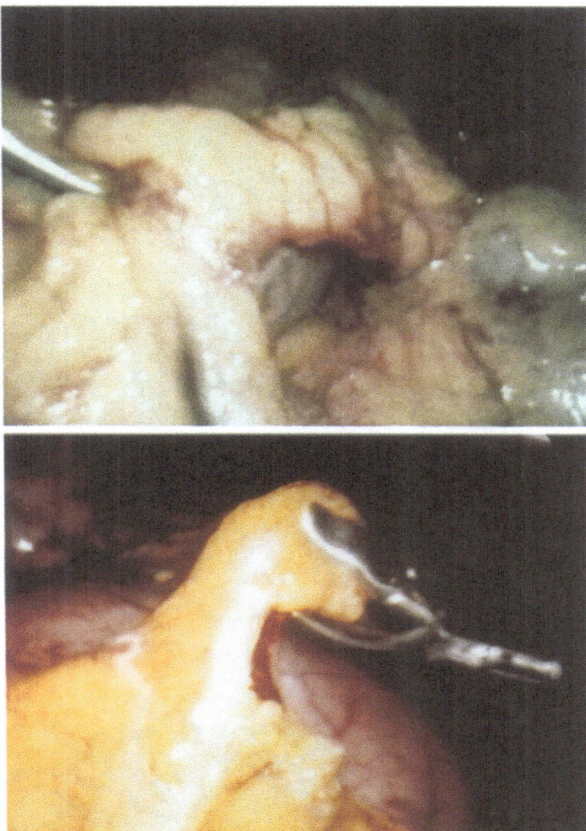

Using this technique we have evaluated 442 consecutive patients with pancreatic and periampullary malignancies between December 1992 and December 1996 at Memorial Sloan-Kettering Cancer Center [28]. After radiological assessment including dynamic CT scan in all patients, 339 (77%) patients were thought to be potentially resectable, 52 (12%) were noted to be unresectable, and 51 (12%) had equivocal findings. Of the 339 patients thought to have resectable disease, 303 patients underwent extended laparoscopic staging as described. Laparoscopic staging identified 48 patients with hepatic metastasis, 41 with extrapancreatic disease, 20 with nodal disease, and another 37 with vascular invasion. After laparoscopic assessment, 199 patients were deemed resectable, and of these 181 (91%) were resected. Only nine patients (19%) were not resected after undergoing laparotomy. In this series laparoscopic assessment provided a positive predictive index of 100%, a negative predictive index of 91%, and an accuracy of 94%.

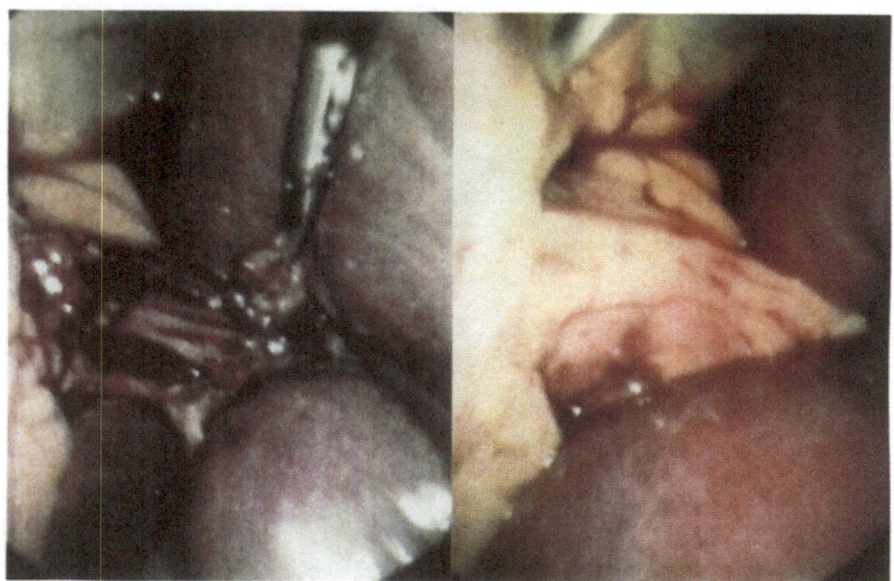

Fig. 6. Laparoscopic hepatic artery lymph node

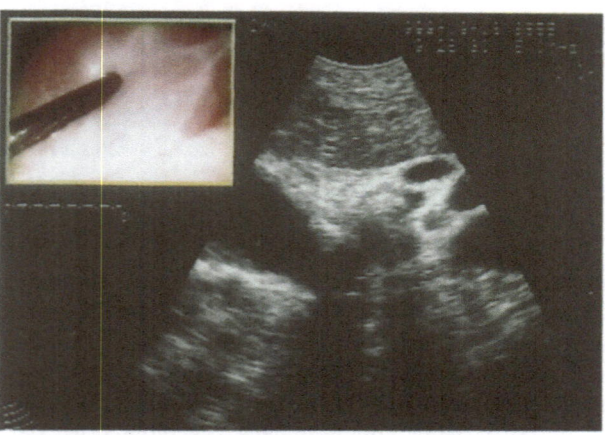

Fig. 7. Laparoscopic ultrasound

Fig. 8. Laparoscopic US of vessels. Schema for evaluating celiac and superior mesenteric axis
CLK Lymph node, *T* tumor, *Dp* pancreactic dvct, *Ao* Aorta, *Du* duodenum, *Lc* candate liver lobe, *Dc* ductus choledochus, *Vp* portal vein

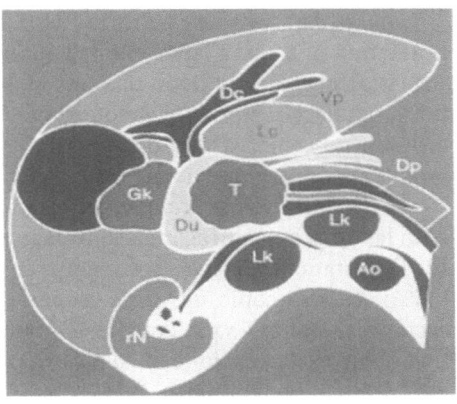

Laparoscopic Ultrasound

Laparoscopic ultrasound is an integral part of the noteworthy improvement achieved in resectability after laparoscopic staging. Laparoscopy alone is limited by being a two-dimensional assessment, such that intraparenchymal liver metastasis deep below the surface and retropancreatic vascular involvement may still be overlooked. Several authors have examined the use of laparoscopic ultrasound in conjunction with laparoscopic staging [20, 21, 23, 29, 30].

Our initial experience with laparoscopic ultrasound demonstrated the utility of this modality and prompted a prospective study of 90 patients with peripancreatic malignancy [20]. Comparing conventional CT imaging, laparoscopic assessment alone, and laparoscopic assessment combined with laparoscopic ultrasound, this study demonstrated 98% accuracy at predicting resectability for the combined approach. A single false positive was noted, providing a positive predictive index of 100% and a negative predictive index of 98%.

Callery et al. reported their experience with staging laparoscopy combined with laparoscopic ultrasound in 50 consecutive patients with hepatic and pancreatic malignancies (HPB) [31]. These patients were considered to have resectable tumors by standard radiographic evaluation. After staging laparoscopy with laparoscopic ultrasonography resectable disease was found in only 28 of 50 patients (56%). At laparotomy, 26 of 28 patients were actually resectable: the false-negative rate was 4%. Staging laparoscopy with laparoscopic ultrasonography indicated unresectability in 22 patients (44%). Staging laparoscopy alone demonstrated previously unrecognized occult metastases in 11 patients (22%). In 11 other patients (22%) in whom staging laparoscopy alone was negative, laparoscopic ultrasonography established unresectability from vascular invasion ($n=5$), lymph node metastases ($n=5$), or intraparenchymal hepatic tumor ($n=1$). The authors suggest that unnecessary laparotomy can be safely avoided by laparoscopic staging with laparoscopic ultrasound in many patients with HPB malignancies, reducing costs and morbidity.

Similar data was also reported by John et al., who performed a prospective evaluation of staging laparoscopy with laparoscopic ultrasonography in predicting surgical resectability in patients with carcinomas of the pancreatic head and periampullary region [21]. A cohort of 40 consecutive patients referred to a tertiary referral center with a diagnosis of potentially resectable pancreatic or periampullary cancer underwent staging laparoscopy with laparoscopic ultrasonography. The diagnostic accuracy of staging laparoscopy alone and in conjunction with laparoscopic ultrasonography was evaluated in predicting tumor resectability. Metastatic lesions were demonstrated by staging laparoscopy in 14 patients (35%). Laparoscopic ultrasonography demonstrated factors confirming unresectable tumor in 23 patients (59%), provided staging information in addition to that of laparoscopy alone in 20 patients (53%), and changed the decision regarding tumor resectability in 10 patients (25%). Staging laparoscopy with laparoscopic ultrasonography was more specific and accurate in predicting tumor resectability than laparoscopy alone (88% and 89% vs. 50% and 65%, respectively). The authors suggest that laparoscopic ultrasonography improves the accuracy of laparoscopic staging in patients with potentially resectable pancreatic and periampullary carcinomas.

Palliative Bypass

Detractors of laparoscopic staging have argued that laparotomy-based staging allows for the creation of prophylactic palliative bypasses for anticipated subsequent biliary or gastric outlet obstruction [32–35]. Prophylactic bypass has been supported by reports that up to 25% of patients would go on to develop gastric outlet obstruction and 70% would develop obstructive jaundice [36–40]. The need for surgical bypass has been to reported to range from 12% to 25% of patients, and historically, bypasses have been routinely performed at the time of the initial exploratory laparotomy [39, 41, 42]. Recently, Van Dijkum et al. reported on 111 patients with peripancreatic disease, 17 of who would have avoided laparotomy by undergoing preoperative laparoscopic staging. However, of these 17 patients, additional open surgery was required in 5 patients, suggesting that the true benefit of laparoscopic staging was only 11% [43].

However, previous reports from our institution have suggested that gastric outlet obstruction occurs in less than 10% of patients with pancreatic adenocarcinoma [13] and surgical palliative bypass procedures carry an unacceptably high rate of complications. In an earlier report from Memorial Sloan-Kettering, postoperative complications following palliative biliary bypass were 18%, following gastroenterostomy 25%, and following exploratory laparotomy alone 12% [13].

The ideal method for achieving palliative biliary decompression remains a topic for discussion; however, at present surgical bypass and endoscopic stenting of the biliary tree are the common approaches [44–46].

Proponents of laparoscopic staging suggest that patients with unresectable disease should undergo nonoperative palliative interventions only when and if they become necessary [35, 47, 48]. Nonoperative interventions such as endoscopic stenting have changed the requirement for open surgery to relieve biliary obstruction in this population [49, 50]. Until recently, the management of patients with malignant obstructive jaundice was almost exclusively surgical; however, multiple reports concerning the use of endoscopic biliary prostheses have demonstrated relief of jaundice and overall survival comparable to patients undergoing surgical bypass [32, 38, 50, 51].

The techniques of laparoscopic biliary bypass and gastroenterostomy have been also been well described [52–55]. This approach may go on to replace open procedures altogether for this patient population, as surgeons gain further experience, because they can be accomplished with shorter recovery time and decreased postprocedure hospital length of stay.

Is There a Role for Prophylactic Bypass?

In a series of 155 consecutive, prospectively followed patients who had undergone laparoscopic staging and were determined to have unresectable pancreatic adenocarcinoma at Memorial Sloan-Kettering Cancer Center, the role for prophylactic biliary or gastric bypass was examined. This group of patients included 40 patients with locally advanced and 115 patients with metastatic disease. Meticulous follow-up demonstrated that only 3% of these patients subsequently required an open operation to treat a malignant obstruction. Although 10% of the patients went on to require biliary decompression, in all cases but one, this was accomplished using endoscopic stents. Only three patients had open gastric bypass performed. These findings suggest that there is a limited role for routine prophylactic bypass in the laparoscopically staged unresectable patient with pancreatic adenocarcinoma. We have recommended that open biliary bypass should be considered only for patients failing endoscopic decompression in the hands of an experienced operator and that gastric bypass should be reserved for those patients with confirmed obstruction [48].

Length of Stay

Patients undergoing laparoscopic staging benefit from a decreased length of hospitalization. We have reported a median hospital stay of 2 days after laparoscopic staging alone [7, 19, 48].

In addition, reduced hospitalization and operative morbidity should translate into decreased delay between surgery and commencement of adjuvant therapy.

Cost of Laparoscopic Staging

The perceived high cost of laparoscopic staging has been an issue for detractors of the technique. Although there are multiple retrospective reports regarding the economic implications of laparoscopic staging, few prospective studies exist. In a prospective study conducted at Memorial Sloan-Kettering Cancer Center be-

Table 1. Advantages of laparoscopic staging in comparison to exploratory laparotomy

A more accurate assessment of resectability than CT alone
Provides accurate clinical staging without exploratory laparotomy
Reduced length of hospitalization compared with laparotomy for staging
Reduced cost of hospitalization for patients staged unresectable before laparotomy
Minimal postoperative delay for the initiation of therapy

tween 1993 and 1995, the total hospital charges for patients with pancreatic cancer undergoing open exploration were compared to those for patients in whom immediate prelaparotomy laparoscopic staging was performed [56] (see Table 1). The results demonstrate a significant reduction in hospital charges for patients with either locally advanced or metastatic disease who underwent an initial laparoscopic staging. Overall, a 25% reduction in total hospital charges was demonstrated in the laparoscopic group. For the main part, these savings were realized by avoiding the cost of unnecessary laparotomy and a reduced length of stay in the hospital [57].

Summary

Laparoscopy for patients with pancreatic cancer provides a minimally invasive procedure with maximum benefits for diagnosis and accurate staging. In comparison to laparotomy, patients undergoing laparoscopy have reduced morbidity, decreased length of hospital stay, and faster return to baseline performance status. Assessment of resectability with more than 90% accuracy is achievable with extended laparoscopy, and in combination with laparoscopic ultrasound even better results have been obtained. Laparoscopic ultrasound is applicable in selected cases particularly when vascular encasement is suggested but not proven by CT. In addition, laparoscopic staging allows for matched cohort neoadjuvant trials to be conducted, as well as a minimal postoperative delay for the initiation of therapy in patients found not to be candidates for resection.

References

1. Brennan MF, Kinsella TJ, Casper ES (1993) Cancer of the Pancreas. In: DeVita VT, Hellman S, Rosenberg SA (eds) Principles and practice of oncology, 5th ed. J.B. Lippincott, Philadelphia, pp 849–882
2. Carter D (1990) Cancer of the Pancreas. Gut 31:494–496
3. Geer R, Brennan M (1993) Resection of Pancreatic Adenocarcinoma: Prognostic Indicators for Survival. Am J Surg 223:279
4. Harrison LE, Brennan MF (1997) Portal vein involvement in pancreatic cancer: a sign of unresectability? Adv Surg 31:375–394

5. Fernandez-del Castillo C, Rattner DW, Warshaw AL (1995) Standards for pancreatic resection in the 1990s. Arch Surg 130:295–299

6. Cameron JL (1995) Long-term survival following pancreaticoduodenectomy for adenocarcinoma of the head of the pancreas. Surg Clin North Am 75:939–951

7. Conlon KC, Dougherty E, Klimstra DS et al (1996) The value of minimal access surgery in the staging of patients with potentially resectable peripancreatic malignancy. Ann Surg 223:134–140

8. Catheline JM, Champault G (1996) Ultrasonic laparoscopy in digestive diseases. Ann Chir 50:51–57

9. Siewert JR, Sendler A, Dittler HJ, Fink U, Hofler H (1995) Staging gastrointestinal cancer as a precondition for multimodal treatment. World J Surg 19:168–177

10. Conlon K, Minnard E (1997) The value of laparoscopic staging in upper gastrointestinal malignancy. The Oncologist 2:10–17

11. Fernandez-del Castillo C, Warshaw AL (1993) Laparoscopy for staging in pancreatic carcinoma. Surg Oncol [Suppl 2] 1:25–29

12. Conlon KC, Klimstra DS, Brennan MF (1996) Long-term survival after curative resection for pancreatic ductal adenocarcinoma. Clinicopathologic analysis of 5-year survivors. Ann Surg 223:273–279

13. de Rooj P, Rogatko A, Brennan M (1991) Evaluation of palliative surgical procedures in unresectable pancreatic cancer. Br J Surg 78:1053–1058

14. Watanapa P, Williamson R (1992) Surgical palliation for pancreatic cancer: Developments during the past two decades. Br J Surg 79:8–20

15. Warshaw AL, Tepper JE, Shipley WU (1986) Laparoscopy in the staging and planning of therapy for pancreatic cancer. Am J Surg 151:76–80

16. Furhman G, Charnsangavej C, Abbruzze J, Martin R, Fenoglio C, Evans D (1994) Thin-section contrast-enhanced computed tomography accurately predicts the resectability of malignant pancreatic neoplasms. Am J Surg 167:104–113

17. Gulliver GM, Baker M, Cheng C (1992) Malignant biliary obstruction: efficacy of thin section dynamic CT scan in determining resectability. Am J Roentgenol Radium Ther Nucl Med 159:503–507

18. Fernandez-del CC, Warshaw AL (1998) Pancreatic cancer. Laparoscopic staging and peritoneal cytology. Surg Oncol Clin North Am 7:135–142

19. Burke EC, Karpeh MS, Conlon KC, Brennan MF (1997) Laparoscopy in the management of gastric adenocarcinoma. Ann Surg 225:262–267

20. Minnard EA, Conlon K, Hoos A, Dougherty E, Hann L, Brennan M (1998) Laparoscopic ultrasound enhances the standard laparoscopy in the staging of pancreatic cancer. Ann Surg 228:1–7

21. John TG, Greig JD, Carter DC, Garden OJ (1995) Carcinoma of the pancreatic head and periampullary region. Tumor staging with laparoscopy and laparoscopic ultrasonography. Ann Surg 221:156–164

22. Holzman M, Reitgen KL, Tyler D, Pappas T (1997) The role of laparoscopy in the management of suspected pancreatic and periampullary malignancies. J Gastrointest Surg 1:236–244

23. Hann LE, Conlon KC, Dougherty EC, Hilton S, Bach AM, Brennan MF (1997) Laparoscopic sonography of peripancreatic tumors: preliminary experience. AJR Am J Roentgenol 169:1257–1262

24. Ishida H (1983) Peritoneoscopy and pancreas biopsy in the diagnosis of pancreatic diseases. Gastrointest Endosc 29:211–218

25. Cuschieri A (1988) Laparoscopy for pancreatic cancer: does it benefit the patient? Eur J Surg Oncol 14:41–44

26. Warshaw AL, Gu ZY, Wittenberg J, Waltman AC (1990) Preoperative staging and assessment of resectability of pancreatic cancer. Arch Surg 125:230–233
27. Harrison LE, Brennan MF (1998) Portal vein resection for pancreatic adenocarcinoma. Surg Oncol Clin North Am 7:165–181
28. Merchant N, Conlon KC (1998) Laparoscopic evaluation in pancreatic cancer. Semin Surg Oncol 15:155–165
29. Murugiah M, Paterson-Brown S, Windsor JA, Miles WF, Garden OJ (1993) Early experience of laparoscopic ultrasonography in the management of pancreatic carcinoma. Surg Endosc 7:177–181
30. Bemelman WA, de WL, van DO et al (1995) Diagnostic laparoscopy combined with laparoscopic ultrasonography in staging of cancer of the pancreatic head region. Br J Surg 82:820–824
31. Callery MP, Strasberg SM, Doherty GM, Soper NJ, Norton JA (1997) Staging laparoscopy with laparoscopic ultrasonography: optimizing resectability in hepatobiliary and pancreatic malignancy. J Am Coll Surg 185:33–39
32. Richards A, Sosin H (1973) Cancer of the pancreas: Value of radical and palliative surgery. Ann Surg 177:325–331
33. Fromm D, Resitarti D, Kozol R (1988) An analysis of when patients eat after gastrojejunostomy. Ann Surg 207:14–20
34. Connie J, Nagpal S, Peebles S (1989) Surgical treatment for adenocarcinoma of the pancreas. Surg Gynecol Obstet 168:437–445
35. Blievernicht SW, Neifeld JP, Terz JJ, Lawrence W Jr (1980) The role of prophylactic gastrojejunostomy for unresectable periampullary carcinoma. Surg Gynecol Obstet 151:794–796
36. Singh S, Longmire W, Reber H (1990) Surgical palliation for pancreatic cancer: The UCLA experience. Ann Surg 212:132–139
37. Warshaw A, Swanson R (1998) Pancreatic Cancer in 1988: Possibilities and probabilities. Ann Surg 208:541–553
38. Potts J, Brougham T, Herman R (1990) Palliative operations for pancreatic carcinoma. Ann Surg 159:72–78
39. Sarr M, Cameron J (1984) Surgical palliation of unresectable carcinoma of the pancreas. World J Surg 8:906–918
40. Meinke W, Twomey PL, Guernsey J, Frey C, Higgings G, Keehn R (1983) Gastric outlet obstruction after palliative surgery for cancer of the head of the pancreas. Arch Surg 118:550–553
41. Hunstad DA, Norton JA (1995) Management of pancreatic carcinoma. Surg Oncol 4:61–74
42. Huguier M, Baumel H, Manderscheild J, Houry S, Fabre J (1993) Surgical palliation for unresected cancer of the exocrine pancreas. Eur J Surg Oncol 19:342–347
43. van Dijkum, EJ, de Witt LT, van Delden OM et al (1997) The efficacy of laparoscopic staging in patients with upper gastrointestinal tumors. Cancer 79:1315–1319
44. Schmassmann A, von GE, Knuchel J, Scheurer U, Fehr HF, Halter (1996) Wallstents versus plastic stents in malignant biliary obstruction: effects of stent patency of the first and second stent on patient compliance and survival. Am J Gastroenterol 91:654–659
45. Vij JC, Govil A, Chaudhary A, Gulati R, Mehta S, Ganguli S (1996) Endoscopic biliary endoprosthesis for palliation of gallbladder carcinoma. Gastroint Endosc 43:121–123
46. Eschelman D, Shapiro M, Bonn J, Sullivan KL, Alden M, Gardiner G (1996) Malignant biliary duct obstruction: Long term experience with Gianturco stents and combined modality radiotherapy. Radiology 200:717–724
47. Schantz S, Schikler W, Evans T, Coffey R (1984) Palliative gastroenterostomy for pancreatic cancer. Am J Surg 147:793–796

48. Espat NJ, Brennan MF, Conlon KC (1999) Laparoscopically staged patients with unresectable pancreatic adenocarcinoma do not require subsequent biliary or gastric bypass. J Am Coll Surg 186: 649–55

49. Friess H, Kleef J, Silva J, Sadowski S, Baer H (1998) The role of diagnostic laparoscopy in pancreatic and periampullary malignancies. J Am Coll of Surg 186:675–682

50. Andersen JR, Sorensen SM, Kruse A, Rokkjaer M, Matzen P (1989) Randomised trial of endoscopic endoprosthesis versus operative bypass in malignant obstructive jaundice. Gut 30:1132–1135

51. Sheperd H, Royle G, Ross A, Diba A, Arthur M, Colin-Jones D (1988) Endoscopic biliary endoprosthesis in the palliation of malignant obstruction of the distal common bile duct: a randomized trial. Br J Surg 75:1166–1168

52. Shimi S, Banting S, Cuschieri A (1992) Laparoscopy in the management of pancreatic cancer: endoscopic cholecystojejunostomy for advanced disease. Br J Surg 79:317–319

53. Fletcher DR, Jones RM (1992) Laparoscopic cholecystjejunostomy as palliation for obstructive jaundice in inoperable carcinoma of pancreas. Surg Endosc 6:147–149

54. Hawasli A (1992) Laparoscopic cholecysto-jejunostomy for obstructing pancreatic cancer: technique and report of two cases. J Laparoendosc Surg 2:351–355

55. Wilson R, Varma J (1992) Laparoscopic gastroenterostomy for malignant duodenal obstruction. Br J Surg 79:1348–1352

56. JarnaginW-R, Conlon K, Bodniewicz J, Dougherty E, DeMatteo R-P, Blumgart L-H, Fong Y (2001) A clinical scoring system predicts the yield of diagnostic laparoscopy in patients with potentially resectable hepatic colorectal metastases. Cancer 91: 1121–8.

57. Jarnagin W-R, Bodniewicz J, Dougherty E, Conlon K, Blumgart L-H, Fong Y (2000) A prospective analysis of staging laparoscopy in patients with primary and secondary hepatobiliary malignancies. J Gastrointest Surg. 4: 34–43.

Laparoscopic Ultrasonography for Staging of Gastrointestinal Cancer

M. Hünerbein · B. Rau · P. Hohenberger · P.M. Schlag

Introduction

Despite the availability of various modern imaging techniques, preoperative staging of gastrointestinal tumors is frequently incorrect. Small intra-abdominal metastases, i.e., liver and lymph node metastases, and peritoneal deposits may not be visualized because of the limited resolution of transcutaneous ultrasonography and computed tomography (CT). Furthermore, accurate assessment of resectability remains a challenge. In recent years, laparoscopy has increasingly been used for staging of gastrointestinal tumors. Recently, the promising results of this technique have been reviewed by several authors [1–3].

However, laparoscopy is not a new technique. More than 10 years ago the value of laparoscopy in detecting unsuspected intra-abdominal tumor spread was well documented by Cuschieri and coworkers [4]. In an early study involving 369 patients with cancer of the esophagus and cardia, laparoscopy revealed metastastic disease in 52 patients [5]. The rate of false negative findings in the patients undergoing subsequent laparotomy ($n=250$) was 4%.

Recent studies have confirmed that laparoscopic inspection of the abdominal cavity offers greater accuracy in the detection of intra-abdominal tumor spread than current-generation CT [6–8]. One major limitation of staging laparoscopy is the lack of tactile information, which restricts the detection of non-superficial lesions such as intraparenchymal liver lesions, lymph node metastases, and retroperitoneal tumor infiltration. Among surgeons there is general agreement that visual assessment alone does not allow evaluation of the curability and resectability of gastrointestinal tumors accurately.

It has been shown that intraoperative ultrasonography is capable of providing information in addition to preoperative staging in patients with primary or secondary liver tumors that can lead to modification of the surgical approach [9]. After the positive experience with intraoperative ultrasonography in open surgery it was a logical consequence to combine the advantages of this technique with a minimally invasive surgical approach.

▌Equipment

In the meantime, specialized equipment was designed for laparoscopic ultra-sonography. Compact ultrasound units were developed that can be placed on the laparoscopy rack, thus saving space in the operating room. The image quality and technical capabilities of these systems are comparable to those of conventional ultrasound units. Various modules, e.g., color Doppler, can be incorporated. New systems can be adjusted and operated by the surgeon with a remote control. The control unit contains all functions that are needed during surgery including measurement, gain adjustment, video activation, and printing. Additional personnel to operate the ultrasound scanner are not necessary. The software allows superimposition of camera images onto ultrasound images or vice versa. All visual information can be displayed on one screen, which facilitates assessment of laparoscopic real-time ultrasonography (Fig. 1). Remote control and transducers are completely immersible for disinfection and can be sterilized by ethylene oxide (<52°C). Alternatively, the instruments can be placed in a sterile cover (Fig. 2).

Second-generation laparoscopic ultrasound probes incorporate high-resolution transducers that can be operated with multiple frequencies (usually 5, 6.5, and 7.5 MHz). The probes have dynamic focus extension ranging from approximately 6 to 90 mm and linear or curved arrays (sector angle 60°). Most probes now have flexible tips that allow bending of the transducer in two directions from +90° to –90° (Fig. 3). However, there are also probes with four degrees of freedom. Flexible instruments facilitate reaching all areas of the abdominal cavity

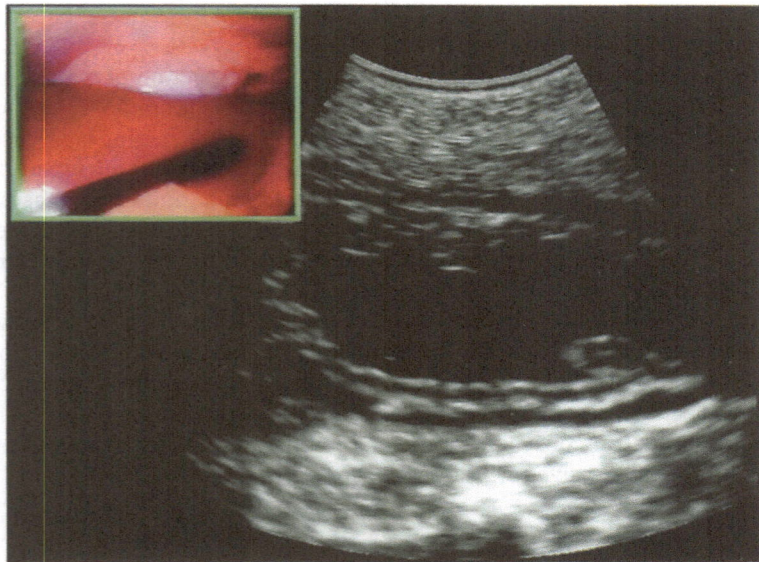

Fig. 1. Picture-in-picture display of laparoscopy and laparoscopic ultrasonography of and stomach liver

without changing the trocar site of the probe. Usually the diameter of the device is approximately 9 mm so that the instrument can be passed through a 10-mm trocar.

Fig. 2. The sterilized remote control for the ultrasound unit enables the surgeon to program the image parameters

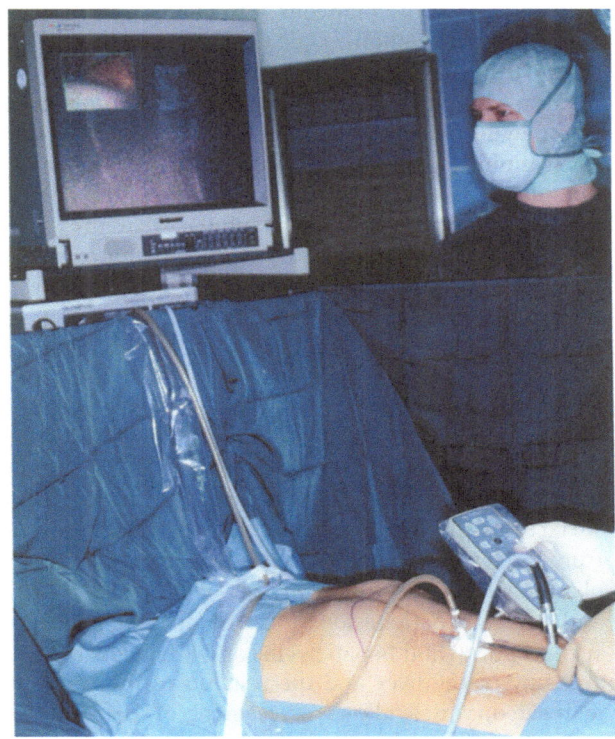

Fig. 3. Laparoscopic ultrasound probe (diameter 9 mm) with a flexible tip and a 5- to 7.5-MHz transducer

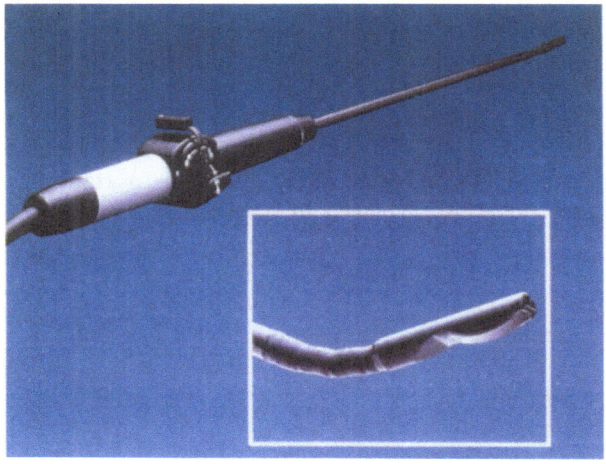

Examination Technique

Laparoscopic ultrasonography must be performed in a systematic way to avoid missing subtle pathology. The intra-abdominal examination follows the same principles as transcutaneous ultrasonography. Nevertheless, special aspects of the technique of laparoscopic ultrasonography have been described [10, 11].

The transducer is usually introduced through a 10-mm port in the right upper quadrant in the anterior axillary line. Depending on the area of interest the position may be changed to another trocar. Generally, the contact technique is used for scanning of solid organs such as the liver. Sometimes a better image quality is obtained by indirect scanning through saline solution. The advantage of this method is that compression of tubular structures such as vessels and gut can be avoided. This method improves the discrimination of the individual wall layers. Furthermore, superficial lesions can be visualized with higher resolution in the focal zone of the transducer.

Ultrasonography of the liver is performed through the left subcostal trocar. The tranducer is placed directly on the left or right liver lobe. The liver is scanned systematically by moving the probe over all segments. The caudal parts of the liver should be examined from both the anterior and posterior surfaces. This is important because small lesions just under the liver capsule can be easily missed because of their close proximity to the transducer. Ultrasonography from both surfaces of the liver can overcome this problem by distancing the transducer from the lesions. In some cases adequate views of segments 7 and 8 can only be obtained from the trocar in the right upper quadrant. Localization, number, and size of hepatic lesions must be documented. Relevant anatomic structures such as portal and hepatic veins and bile ducts can be visualized. The segmental anatomy of the liver and the relation of the tumor to these structures can be delineated, which allows assessment of the extent of the resection and the amount and function of the remaining liver tissue [12]. The structures of the porta hepatis can be best assessed (longitudinal section) when the probe is introduced through the left subcostal trocar and placed on segment 4 of the liver. The distal part of the common bile duct is identified by positioning the transducer directly on the hepatoduodenal ligament. The stomach can be visualized by direct contact scanning or using the liver as an acoustic window. Acoustic shadowing of the posterior wall of the stomach and the pancreas can be avoided by instillation of 300–500 ml of saline solution through a nasogastric tube into the stomach. The branches of the celiac axis, portal vein, superior mesenteric artery, and aorta are displayed in transverse sections from the left subcostal trocar. Lymph nodes along these vessels are classified according to the TNM classification of the UICC as N1, N2, or distant metastases. Metastatic lymph node involvement is characterized by hypoechoic pattern, round shape, well-demarcated boundaries and a size of more than 1 cm. Color Doppler examinations can be helpful to delineate vascular anatomy and to distinguish vessels from lymph nodes (Fig. 4).

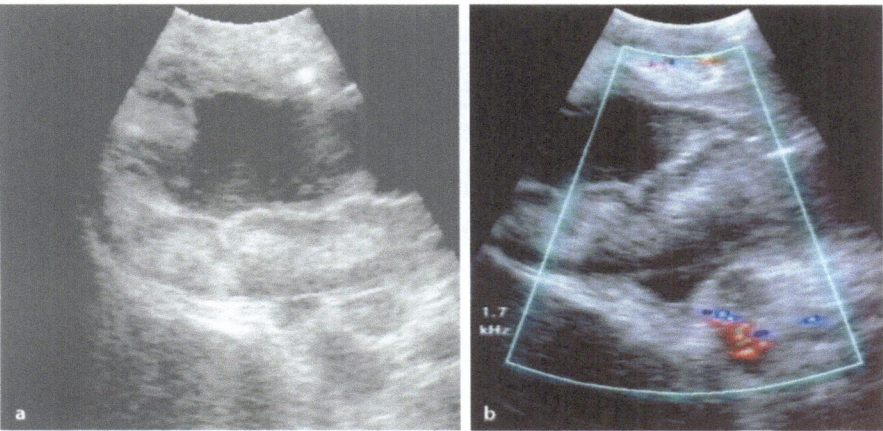

Fig. 4a, b. Laparoscopic ultrasonography of gastric cancer (T2) and perigastric lymph nodes without (a) and with color Doppler (b)

Results

Gastroesophageal Cancer

Local staging of esophageal and gastric cancer has been significantly improved by endoscopic ultrasonography (EUS). However, reliable assessment of distant metastases, i.e., liver metastases, peritoneal carcinosis and spread to extraregional lymph nodes cannot be obtained by EUS. Therefore, EUS often fails to provide a correct diagnosis in patients with advanced tumors. Accurate determination of resectability remains a challenge in patients with gastric cancer.

In a comparative study Watt et al investigated the accuracy of laparoscopy, CT, and transcutaneous ultrasonography in detecting intra-abdominal metastases in 90 patients with esophageal or gastric carcinoma [13]. Laparoscopy showed a sensitivity of 89% in the diagnosis of peritoneal metastases, whereas ultrasound and CT reached a sensitivity of 22% and 0%, respectively. Laparoscopy was more sensitive for hepatic metastases (96%) than either ultrasound (48%), or CT (56%). Figure 5 shows a small hepatic metastasis that was only detected by laparoscopic ultrasonography.

To date, only a limited number of studies have been performed in which the role of laparoscopic ultrasonography for staging of esophageal and gastric cancer was investigated systematically. Most authors have reported their cumulative experience and have not differentiated between esophageal and gastric cancer. Anderson et al. prospectively compared laparoscopy with ultrasonography to conventional preoperative imaging in 43 patients with gastroesophageal cancer [14]. Because of the findings at laparoscopy, resection was abandoned in 6 of 43 patients who were regarded as having resectable disease by transcutaneous ultrasonography and CT. This was because of peritoneal deposits (n=4), liver metastases (n=1) and extensive local disease. The exclusion of these patients resulted in

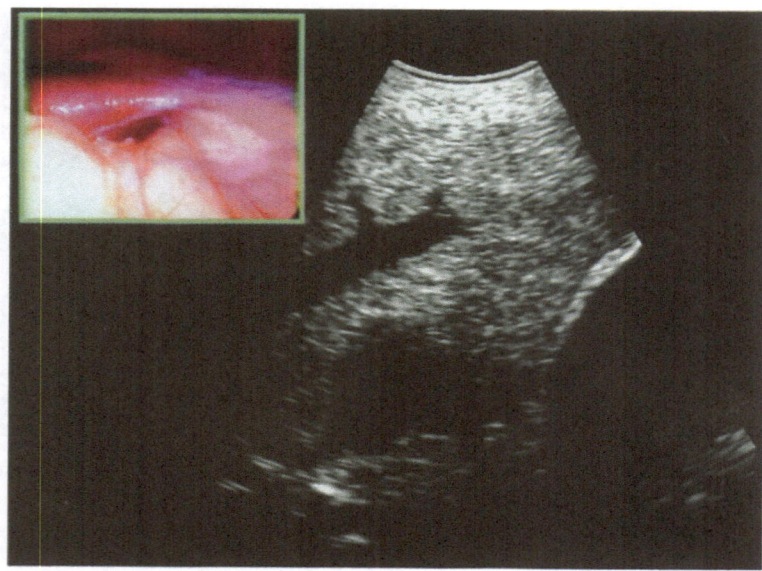

Fig. 5. Laparoscopic ultrasonography of the liver with a hypoechoic liver metastasis in segment 5 near the gallbladder

a resection rate of 97% compared with 79% for conventional staging. Laparoscopic ultrasonography improved the evaluation of local tumor infiltration and lymph node involvement and disclosed a liver metastases that was not detected with other staging modalities. However, no other patients were excluded from surgical exploration on the basis of laparoscopic ultrasonography. In a group of 92 patients with gastric cancer, Conlon et al. [15] found metastatic disease unappreciated by conventional staging modalities in 31 patients. In their experience, the addition of laparoscopic ultrasonography to laparoscopy increased the accuracy of M1 screening and introduced T and N staging capabilities.

Recently, Finch et al. performed a detailed analysis of the value of laparoscopic ultrasonography in 26 patients with gastroesophageal cancer [7]. Resectability for potential cure was determined by means of CT, laparoscopy, and laparoscopic ultrasound with accuracies of 68%, 88%, and 96%, respectively. Overall staging of metastases was 70% accurate for CT versus 84% for laparoscopy and 92% for laparoscopic ultrasonography. Laparoscopic ultrasonography provided additional information with clinical relevance in all 23 patients. This included 24 items of positive information and 87 items of negative information. In another prospective study of 56 patients, it seemed that the major benefit of combined laparoscopic staging was for patients with lesions of the lower esophagus and the gastric cardia [16]. Laparoscopic staging resulted in a change in stage in 41% of all cases and in only 6% of the patients with middle third esophageal cancer.

We have analyzed the impact of staging laparoscopy with ultrasonography in 134 consecutive patients with gastric cancer [17]. Statistical analysis showed a

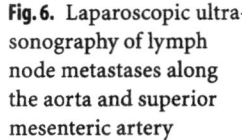

Fig. 6. Laparoscopic ultra-sonography of lymph node metastases along the aorta and superior mesenteric artery

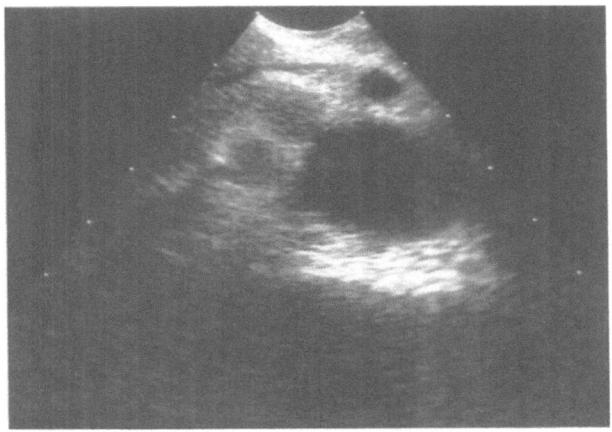

significantly ($p<0.01$) better accuracy for laparoscopy in the detection of distant metastases (92%) than for transcutaneous ultrasound (63%) or computed tomography (58%). Incurable disease was identified in 48 patients (36%). False negative results were only obtained in five cases because of minimal peritoneal seeding ($n=2$), M1 lymph nodes ($n=1$), and nonresectable disease ($n=2$).

In our experience, laparoscopic ultrasonography was very useful to guide laparoscopic excision of distant lymph nodes for histopathological analysis (Fig. 6).

According to data in the literature, laparoscopic staging is indicated for all patients with nonobstructed, nonbleeding gastric adenocarcinoma, except early gastric cancer. With respect to multimodal therapy it seems reasonable to perform staging laparoscopy in patients with squamous cell carcinoma of the distal esophagus and adenocarcinoma of the cardia.

Pancreatic Cancer

Despite the advent of ultrafast MRI, accurate evaluation of distant metastases and local resectability in pancreatic cancer remains difficult. It has already been demonstrated that laparoscopy is capable of improving the diagnosis of intra-abdominal metastases in patients with pancreatic cancer, thus avoiding unnecessary laparotomy. Almost 10 years ago Warshaw et al. [18] published the results of staging laparoscopy in 40 patients with pancreatic cancer. Fourteen patients had positive findings during laparoscopy. However, liver metastases were found in a further 3 of the 26 patients who underwent subsequent laparotomy. In another early study [4] 42 of 51 patients were correctly staged as having nonresectable disease by laparoscopy. Nevertheless, only four of the nine patients considered resectable were resected. Some surgeons have questioned the value of staging laparoscopy in pancreatic cancer because accurate assessment of local resectability is limited by the lack of tactile sensation.

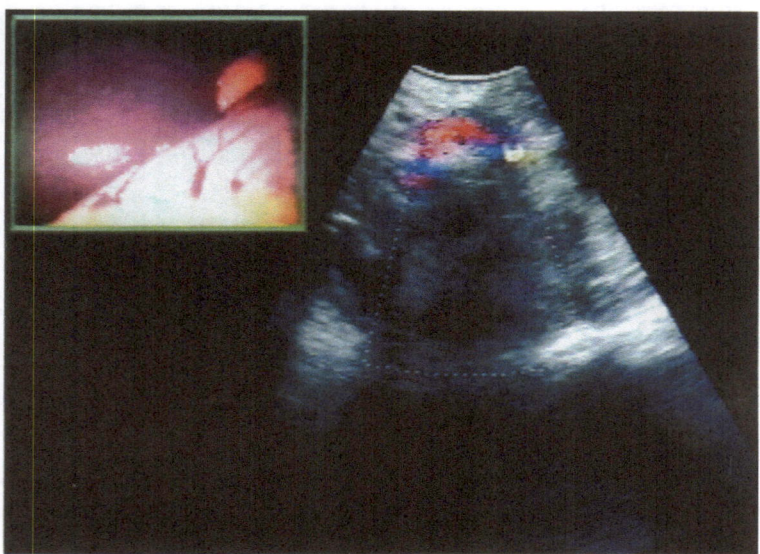

Fig. 7. Laparoscopic color Doppler ultrasonography of a hypoechoic pancreatic carcinoma with close relation to the portal vein indicating nonresectable disease

Nonresectable disease can be assumed in the presence of one of the following factors (histological confirmation): (1) extrapancreatic infiltration (e.g., mesocolon); (2) involvement of celiac or high portal lymph nodes; (3) invasion or entrapment of the celiac axis, hepatic artery, or superior mesenteric artery. Extended resections may be indicated in selected patients with involvement of the portal or mesenteric vein (Fig. 7).

All the factors mentioned above can be readily identified by laparoscopic ultrasound, especially when color Doppler capabilities are available. Recently, it was demonstrated that the vascular structures can be accurately visualized by laparoscopic ultrasonography in approximately 95% of patients [19]. In this study a complete laparoscopic examination including ultrasonography was performed in 90 patients with tumors in the head of the pancreas. The positive predictive index, negative predictive index, and accuracy of laparoscopy with the addition of ultrasonography in the determination of resectability were 100%, 98%, and 98%, respectively. In another study involving 70 patients with carcinoma of the pancreatic head region, the role of combined laparoscopic staging for local and overall nonresectability was investigated [16]. Metastatic spread was correctly diagnosed in 16 of 21 patients; laparoscopic ultrasonography revealed 2 additional liver metastases. On the basis of ultrasonography, local resectability was assumed in 22 tumors, 21 of which were subsequently resected. The positive and negative predictive values for local nonresectability were 93% and 74%, respectively. The corresponding figures for local nonresectability and metastatic disease were 97% and 65%.

John et al. [20] published a detailed study on the value of laparoscopic ultrasonography in a series of 40 patients with pancreatic cancer. Occult metastatic lesions were demonstrated by laparoscopy in 14 patients. However, laparoscopy alone failed to identify 12 patients with locoregional tumor nonresectability. Intraoperative ultrasonography showed nonresectable tumors in 23 patients and provided relevant staging information in addition to that of laparoscopy in 20 patients (53%). The overall accuracy of combined laparoscopic staging and laparoscopy alone in predicting tumor resectability was 89% and 65%, respectively.

The currently available data on laparoscopic ultrasonography in pancreatic cancer give evidence that this technique enhances the accuracy of staging laparoscopy significantly. This technique must be considered as an integral part of laparoscopic staging of pancreatic cancer.

Once nonresectable disease is diagnosed in patients with pancreatic cancer, palliative treatment must be considered. In the meantime, bypass procedures are increasingly performed laparoscopically [21], which makes accurate laparoscopic staging including intraoperative ultrasonography even more important.

Hepatic Metastases and Hepatocellular Carcinoma

The presence of metastatic spread to the liver precludes curative resection of most primaries. For selected patients with primary or secondary liver tumors, aggressive liver resection provides the only realistic chance for long-term survival. However, this is a controversial issue, and careful patient selection is crucial to obtain good outcome of the patients. Multifocal liver metastases and extrahepatic dissemination such as nodal spread and peritoneal carcinosis are considered a contraindication to liver resection.

Until now the most sensitive method for staging of primary and secondary liver tumors has been a combination of careful open palpation and intraoperative ultrasonography. Several studies have confirmed the superiority of this approach to conventional preoperative imaging. In the meantime, several studies have been performed to investigate the feasibility of intraoperative liver ultrasonography via a laparoscopic approach.

John and coworkers examined the impact of laparoscopic ultrasonography on the assessment of resectability in 43 patients with potentially resectable liver tumors [1]. Laparoscopy demonstrated factors precluding curative resection in 46% of the patients. Among these laparoscopic ultrasonography identified liver tumors not visible during laparoscopy in 14 patients (33%). The resectability rate was significantly higher among those patients undergoing laparoscopic staging (93%) compared with those in whom primary laparoscopy was performed (58%).

In the last years there has been growing interest in laparoscopic colectomy for colorectal cancer. Precise laparoscopic staging is of paramount importance for laparoscopic colorectal surgery, because subsequent laparotomy and liver palpation are not performed. However, there is a lack of systematic studies evaluating the accuracy of laparoscopic staging during laparoscopic surgery for colorectal cancer. Marchesa et al. [22] prospectively studied the accuracy of laparoscopy in

22 patients, who underwent laparoscopy for resection of colorectal cancer. In seven patients laparoscopic ultrasonography and preoperative CT identified 16 and 10 lesions, respectively. In one patient detection of an unsuspected metastasis by ultrasonography led to conversion to laparotomy. Wedge liver resection was performed after biopsy confirmation of a metastasis. Another study compared the accuracy of laparoscopic liver ultrasound with open intraoperative ultrasound and palpation in colorectal cancer. In experimental and clinical examinations three pig livers with 18 lesions and 15 patients were studied. The sensitivity and specificity of laparoscopy were 94% and 78% in the animal study and 80% and 91% in the human study [23].

Major hepatic resections may be performed in patients with hepatocellular carcinoma (HCC), because no other treatment offers the chance for long-term survival. Selection of patients for curative hepatic resection involves accurate assessment of the extent of disease. Furthermore, it is crucial to determine the extent of resection and the hepatic reserve. Lo et al. [24] analyzed the value of laparoscopic ultrasonography in 91 patients with HCC who were considered candidates for curative resection. In 15 of these patients laparoscopy revealed nonresectable disease because of metastatic spread, intravascular tumor thrombi, invasion into adjacent organs and inadequate liver remnant. Among the remaining 76 patients who underwent laparotomy, 9 had exploration only and 67 were resected.

In summary, the advantages of intraoperative ultrasonography in the assessment of patients under consideration for hepatic resection can be obtained by a minimally invasive approach.

▮ Summary

There is evidence that laparoscopy is more accurate in the detection of intra-abdominal metastases than conventional preoperative imaging (Table 1). However, it is obvious that laparoscopic inspection of the abdominal cavity is not adequate for the detection of deep-seated liver metastases and lymph node metastases. Therefore, laparoscopic ultrasound is an ideal adjunct to laparoscopy, because this technique may compensate the lack of tactile feedback with laparoscopic instruments. This is of major importance for the assessment of occult liver metastases and lymph node involvement. Color-coded Doppler imaging can be very valuable for the assessment resectability in patients with pancreatic cancer. Current data confirm that laparoscopic ultrasound is capable of enhancing the accuracy of staging laparoscopy. Compared with standard laparoscopy, the combination of both techniques increases the sensitivity of staging laparoscopy in the determination of nonresectable disease markedly (Table 2). Laparoscopic ultrasonography must be considered as an integral part of staging laparoscopy.

Table 1. Comparative accuracy of conventional staging (CT/US), staging laparoscopy (LAP), and laparoscopic ultrasonography (LAPUS) in the detection of intra-abdominal metastases in gastric cancer

Author	Year	n	Accuracy CT/US	LAP	LAPUS
D'Ugo [8]	1996	70	74%	100%	–
Stell [25]	1996	103	60%	75%	
Finch [7]	1997	26	70%	84%	92%
Hünerbein [17]	1998	134	45%		93%

Table 2. Comparative sensitivity of laparoscopy (LAP) and laparoscopic ultrasonography (LAPUS) in the detection of nonresectable disease

Author	Year	Tumor	n	LAP	LAPUS
Bemelman [16]	1995	Pancreas	70	67%	72%
John [20]	1995	Pancreas	40	65%	89%
Callery [26]	1997	Pancreas	50	45%	92%
Minnard [27]	1998	Pancreas	90	72%	98%
John [1]	1994	Liver	50	62%	86%
Ramijn [28]	1998	Gastroesophageal	60	31%	81%

References

1. John TG, Garden OJ (1994) Laparoscopic ultrasonography: extending the scope of diagnostic laparoscopy. Br J Surg 81:5–6
2. Thompson DM, Arregui ME (1998) Role of laparoscopic ultrasound in cancer management. Semin Surg Oncol 15:166–175
3. Conlon KCP, Minnard EA (1997) The value of laparoscopic staging in upper gastrointestinal malignancy. Oncologist 2:10–17
4. Cuschieri A (1988) Laparoscopy for pancreatic cancer: does it benefit the patient. Eur J Surg Oncol 14:41–44
5. Dagini G, Caldironi MW, Marin G (1986) Laparoscopy in abdominal staging of esophageal cancer. Gastrointest Endosc 32:400–402
6. Hünerbein M, Rau B, Schlag PM (1995) Laparoscopy and laparoscopic ultrasound for staging of upper gastrointestinal tumours. Eur J Surg Oncol 21:50–55
7. Finch MD, John TG, Garden OJ et al (1997) Laparoscopic ultrasonography for staging gastroesophageal cancer. Surgery 121:10–17
8. D'Ugo DM, Coppola R, Persiani R et al (1996) Immediately preoperative laparoscopic staging for gastric cancer. Surg Endosc 10:996–999
9. Ravikumar TS (1996) Laparoscopic staging and intraoperative ultrasonography for liver tumor management. Surg Oncol Clin North Am 5:271–281

10. Machi J, Schwartz JH, Zaren HA et al (1996) Technique of laparoscopic ultrasound examination of the liver and pancreas. Surg Endoscopy 10:684–689

11. van Delden OM, de Wit LT, Bemelman WA et al (1997) Laparoscopic ultrasonography for abdominal tumor staging: technical aspects and imaging findings. Abdom Imaging 22:125–131

12. Yamamoto M, Stiegmann GV, Durham J et al (1993) Laparoscopy guided intracorporeal ultrasound accurately delineates hepatobiliary anatomy. Surg Endosc 7:325–330

13. Watt J, Stewart J, Anderson D et al (1989) Laparoscopy, ultrasound and computed tomography in cancer of the esophagus and gastric cardia: a prospective comparison for detecting intra-abdominal metastases. Br J Surg 76:1036–1039

14. Anderson DN, Campbell S, Park KGM (1996) Accuracy of laparoscopic ultrasonography in the staging of upper gastrointestinal malignancy. Br J Surg 83:1424–1428

15. Conlon KC, Karpeh MSJ (1996) Laparoscopy and laparoscopic ultrasound in the staging of gastric cancer. Semin Oncol 23:347–351

16. Bemelmann WA, de Wit LT, van Delden OM (1995) Diagnostic laparoscopy combined with laparoscopic ultrasonography in staging of cancer of the pancreatic head region. Br J Surg 82:820–824

17. Hünerbein M, Rau B, Hohenberger P, Schlag PM (1998) The role of staging laparoscopy for multimodal therapy of gastrointestinal cancer. Surg Endoscopy 12:921–925

18. Warshaw AL, Gu ZY, Wittenberg J, Waltman AC (1990) Preoperative staging and assessment of resectability of pancreatic cancer. Arch Surg 125:230–233

19. Merchant NB, Conlon KC (1998) Laparoscopic evaluation in pancreatic cancer. Semin Surg Oncol 15:155–156

20. John TG, Greig JD, Carter DC, Garden OJ (1995) Carcinoma of the pancreatic head and periampullary region. Tumor staging with laparoscopy and laparoscopic ultrasonography. Ann Surg 221:156–164

21. Rau B, Hünerbein M, Schlag PM (1996) Advantages of laparoscopic palliative surgery in upper GI tract cancer. Cancer Treat Rev 22 (Suppl A):109–111

22. Marchesa P, Milsom JW, Hale JC et al (1996) Intraoperative laparoscopic liver ultrasonography for staging of colorectal cancer. Dis Colon Rectum 39:S73–S78

23. Foley EF, Kolecki RV, Schirmer BD (1998) The accuracy of laparoscopic ultrasound in the detection of colorectal cancer liver metastases. Am J Surg 176:262–264

24. Lo CM, Lai ECS, Liu CL et al (1998) Laparoscopy and laparoscopic ultrasonography avoid exploratory laparotomy in patients with hepatocellular carcinoma. Ann Surg 227:527–532

25. Stell DA, Carter CR, Stewart I, Anderson JR (1996) Prospective comparison of laparoscopy, ultrasonography and computed tomography in the staging of gastric cancer. Br J Surg 83:1260–1262

26. Callery MP, Strasberg SM, Doherty GM et al (1997) Staging laparoscopy with laparoscopic ultrasonography: optimizing resectability in hepatobiliary and pancreatic malignancy. J Am Coll Surg 185:33–39

27. Minnard EA, Conlon KC, Hoos A et al (1998) Laparoscopic ultrasound enhances standard laparoscopy in the staging of pancreatic cancer. Ann Surg 228:182–187

28. Romijn MG, van Overhagen H, Spillenaar Bilgen EJ et al (1998) Laparoscopy and laparoscopic ultrasonography in staging of oesophageal and cardial carcinoma. Br J Surg 85:1010–1012

Further Results and Strategies
of Clinical Application

Contribution to Initial Staging and Assessment of Treatment Results in Gynecologic Cancers

J.P. CURTIN

Overview

Laparoscopic surgery has long been associated with gynecologic procedures, and the more recent introduction of videolaparoscopy has expanded the indications for laparoscopically assisted procedures for both benign and malignant conditions of the female genital tract. In the United States, approximately 70,000–80,000 new cases of invasive gynecologic cancers were diagnosed in 1999. The most common gynecologic cancer is endometrial cancer (37,400 cases/year), followed by ovarian cancer (25,200 cases/year) and cervical cancer (12,800 cases/year) [1]. For the majority of women with these conditions, surgery is the initial mode of treatment. For each of the major sites of gynecologic cancer, the role of laparoscopic surgery continues to develop. In this chapter, the current status of laparoscopic surgery for gynecologic neoplasms, as well as our institutional experience with this approach, will be explored.

Ovarian Neoplasms

Assessment of ovarian neoplasms is one of the most extensively described topics in the field of gynecologic laparoscopic surgery. Overall, the majority of reports in the literature focus on the potential risks and benefits of the laparoscopic management of adnexal masses. Historically, laparoscopy has been used to manage patients with known ovarian cancer for two purposes: in the pretreatment evaluation of patients whose initial laparotomy was felt to be inadequate; and as a „second-look" procedure to preclude laparotomy in patients with persistent disease after primary chemotherapy. A more recent application is the complete laparoscopic staging of apparent early-stage disease.

Adnexal Mass

Evaluation and treatment of the woman with an adnexal mass is a common clinical problem. A review of more than 5 million hospitalizations of reproductive-age women for gynecologic disorders in the United States during a 3-year period

(1988–1990) found that ovarian cysts were the second most prevalent discharge diagnosis, representing 10% of the total number of patients studied [2]. In addition to normal physiological ovarian enlargement, there is an extensive list of neoplastic and tumor-like conditions that can arise in the ovary. Frequently, the correct diagnosis can only be established by pathological examination after surgical removal of the adnexal mass. When surgical management is chosen, the primary concern is the exclusion of a malignant neoplasm; the secondary benefits are relief of symptoms, diagnosis and treatment of endometriosis, and preservation of ovarian function. There is considerable debate as to whether removal of the common benign ovarian neoplasms (e.g., serous cystadenoma) represents removal of a premalignant lesion and prevention of ovarian cancer.

The revolution in minimal access surgery has also had a major impact on the management of the patient with an adnexal mass. Given that approximately 80% of all ovarian neoplasms are benign, most women are candidates for a laparoscopic approach when surgery is indicated for an adnexal mass. Although minimal-access surgery has the advantage of shorter hospitalization and a more rapid resumption of normal activities, it remains a major surgical procedure; the capability of doing a laparoscopic procedure should not promote a more liberal approach to the surgical evaluation of the woman with an adnexal mass.

Preoperative Evaluation

Serum Ca-125

The quantitative measurement of the serum level of the antigen Ca-125 can be an important component of the decision-making process in the management of the patient with a suspected adnexal mass. First described by Bast and colleagues in 1983 [3], Ca-125 is a glycoprotein produced by a variety of normal as well as neoplastic tissue. The established upper limit of normal serum Ca-125 levels ranges from 25–35 U/ml. The current accepted clinical indications for serum Ca-125 measurement include preoperative evaluation of the patient with a suspected ovarian neoplasm and monitoring of patients with an established diagnosis of ovarian cancer.

As a preoperative test for the woman with an ovarian neoplasm, Ca-125 levels are helpful in predicting whether the mass is benign or malignant. When other clinical factors, including the clinical impression of the pelvic mass, ultrasonic characteristics, and the presence or absence of ascites, are combined with serum Ca-125 determinations, Ca-125 will improve both the positive and negative predictive value of pathology before surgery; the added sensitivity and specificity is of greater value in the postmenopausal patient, reflecting the higher prevalence of ovarian cancer among women aged 50 years or older [4–6]. The limitations of serum Ca-125 determinations in premenopausal women are related to the prevalence of benign conditions associated with an elevated Ca-125 level, including endometriosis, pregnancy, pelvic inflammatory disease, and uterine leiomyoma.

Ultrasound

The improvement in ultrasound technology and the near universal availability of pelvic and transvaginal ultrasound have had a profound effect on the diagnosis and management of the adnexal mass. In many cases, the sonographic findings are the primary indication for surgery.

The first consideration of the ultrasound examination is to determine whether the pelvic mass is an ovarian mass or whether there is a possibility that the mass arises from another pelvic organ. The ultrasonographer should comment on the ability to image the normal ovary if possible. If the laterality can be determined, this information may be important in obtaining informed consent. In addition to the ovaries, the uterine image should also be noted with comment on any abnormality.

Measurement of the size and the morphological features of the abnormal ovary are the most important ultrasonic determinates guiding the clinical decision-making process. At minimum, a two-dimensional measurement of the largest diameters should be clearly stated; if possible, three dimensions should be measured to allow for the calculation of volume of the mass. If the mass is less than 5 cm in maximum diameter and is a simple cyst without internal echoes, there is a very low incidence of malignancy [7]. In the postmenopausal patient, a mass greater than 5 cm in any dimension, regardless of morphology, is probably a neoplastic lesion.

Given the multiple causes of adnexal enlargement in the premenopausal patient, findings of ovarian enlargement of up to 10 cm in diameter associated with a functional process is not uncommon. Morphology of the premenopausal patient with an enlarged ovary that is less than 10 cm in diameter may also be difficult to interpret because functional cysts, endometriosis, and infectious sequelae may result in a complex ultrasonic appearance, which in a postmenopausal women would be much more ominous. Morphological features that are most worrisome include internal papillary projections and solid masses.

Several scoring systems have been proposed as an adjunct to the standard ultrasound report. For the most part, these scoring systems are effective in their negative predictive value (i.e., predicting benign ovarian mass). In one series by Lerner and colleagues [8], using a morphological scoring system analyzing wall structure, septation, echogenicity, and shadowing, the authors were able to accurately predict a benign process in 247 of 248 (99.7%) patients studied. However, in predicting a malignant process, the scoring systems are less reliable. In part, this may be due to the fact that most patients reported in clinical studies are premenopausal and the vast majority do not have an ovarian cancer [9].

Reproductive-Age Patients

When the diagnosis of an adnexal mass is suspected by history and physical examination in a reproductive-age woman, an ultrasound should be performed to further characterize the mass. For most patients, the differential diagnosis includes a functional cyst versus a benign neoplasm. Surgery should be considered if there is an interval increase in the size or complexity of the mass. Other factors that may influence the decision to operate include a rising serum Ca-125, pain, and/or patient anxiety.

There can be no absolute limitation to the decision to use either laparoscopy or laparotomy; the two surgical methods should be viewed as complimentary rather than competing. A corollary to this concept is that laparoscopy should be viewed as a major surgical procedure and should not be offered as an intermediate to a laparotomy; indications for surgical evaluation should be the same whether the method of surgery is to be laparoscopy or laparotomy. If the premenopausal patient requires surgical evaluation and treatment of an adnexal mass, many patients will be candidates for a laparoscopic procedure. Mini-laparotomy is another alternative to laparotomy [10]. The advantages of either laparoscopy or mini-laparotomy are related to decreased hospitalization, less discomfort, and faster recovery [10, 11]. The general exceptions are patients with very large lesions of the ovary(ies) or patients with an obvious malignant process; these patients will often be candidates for laparotomy. The informed consent document must carefully delineate the planned extent of surgery and outline the limits of acceptable alternatives if there is an unexpected finding during surgery (i.e., ovarian cystectomy versus oophorectomy). Because many laparoscopic procedures for adnexal masses can be safely accomplished in an outpatient surgical center, the assessment of the need to convert electively to an open laparotomy may be best done on another day in an operating suite capable of supporting a more advanced surgical procedure. This two-step method also allows for the proper scheduling of consultant surgeons if needed and permanent pathological review of the surgical specimen.

In a small number of cases, a malignant process will either be confirmed or suspected based on clinical findings and/or frozen-section diagnosis. In large series and surveys, the malignancy rate of adnexal masses managed by laparoscopy is usually less than 5% [12–14]. The decision to proceed with a more extensive surgery must be made carefully. Unless the surgeon is absolutely confident in the frozen-section diagnosis and is capable of performing a complete primary resection of the ovarian neoplasm and a thorough surgical staging, the prudent choice in this situation is to obtain tissue for permanent pathological study and terminate the procedure [15, 16]. In the situation where the patient has a germ cell malignancy or a low-malignant-potential tumor of the ovary and desires retention of reproductive potential, fertility-preserving surgery is generally associated with an equivalent outcome compared with bilateral salpingo-oophorectomy.

Rupture of an ovarian malignancy is a concern when the patient has an early ovarian cancer [17, 18]. Rupture may occur whether the surgical procedure is performed by laparoscopy or laparotomy. The impact on prognosis is debatable. In a small number of patients, rupture of an ovarian malignancy will be the single factor that determines the necessity for adjuvant chemotherapy. In most cases, rupture occurs inadvertently during the surgical procedure. When there is a strong suspicion that an ovarian mass is malignant, planned rupture to facilitate removal should be avoided.

Postmenopausal Patients

When the diagnosis of an adnexal mass is made in a postmenopausal woman and there is a lower suspicion of an ovarian cancer, laparoscopic evaluation can be considered. The criteria for laparoscopic surgery rather than laparotomy are the same as for the younger woman: the mass should be removable by laparoscopic techniques, and there should be a low likelihood that the mass is a malignant process. When a patient has a unilateral adnexal mass and surgery is planned, in most cases a bilateral oophorectomy is performed. In one series, 65 postmenopausal women aged 50 years or older with simple adnexal masses ranging in size from 2 to 10 cm in diameter and normal serum Ca-125 levels underwent an initial laparoscopic procedure [19]. Almost all procedures were successfully completed as a laparoscopic procedure. In this limited series there were no cases of malignancy.

As is true of younger women, when a laparoscopic approach is chosen as the initial method to evaluate a postmenopausal patient with an adnexal mass, the surgeon and the patient should have a clear understanding of the back-up plan in the situation where the patient is found to have an ovarian malignancy. The best alternative is immediate conversion to a laparotomy when the laparoscopic findings confirm an ovarian cancer. Complete laparoscopic management of an ovarian cancer by bilateral oophorectomy, hysterectomy, and extended surgical staging including retroperitoneal lymph node sampling has been reported but must be considered as an unproven surgical method for the treatment of a newly diagnosed ovarian cancer [20].

Indications for surgical removal of an adnexal mass in a postmenopausal patient include an ovarian mass with a maximum diameter of greater than 5 cm, a rising serum Ca-125, and/or development of a complex intracystic echo pattern. The approach and preoperative planning regarding conversion to an open laparotomy should be detailed. As is true for the premenopausal woman, if the laparoscopic surgeon discovers an unsuspected ovarian malignancy and is not prepared for laparotomy and thorough surgical staging, the procedure is best terminated and the patient is best served by referral to the appropriate surgeon.

In a review of the initial Memorial Hospital experience with laparoscopic management of ovarian neoplasms, we had a higher rate of malignancy than is reported in the literature. The overall malignancy rate among the 300 patients reviewed was 13%. The higher than average malignancy rate probably reflects the nature of our referral population, which tends to have a higher number of older women and a significant number of patients previously treated for nongynecologic malignancy. Nearly one-half of the patients with a malignant ovarian neoplasm had a prior history of nongynecologic cancers. As we previously reported, laparoscopy is well suited to the initial evaluation of this subset of patients [21]. Most common cancers metastatic to the ovary include breast, colon, and gastric. If the ovarian neoplasm is a metastatic lesion, laparotomy may still be indicated if the ovarian mass cannot be removed laparoscopically. However, if the laparoscopic evaluation demonstrates intra-abdominal disease, then the procedure can be stopped and the patient is spared a laparotomy. If the patient is found to have an ovarian malignancy, the majority of patients at our institution are then converted to an open laparotomy. It continues to be our recommendation that except for individual cases, most patients with presumed early-stage ovarian cancer diagnosed at laparoscopy will benefit from an open procedure, as the optimal approach for thorough and accurate staging.

▌ Second-Look Laparoscopy

The second-look operation for ovarian carcinoma is the most accurate method of assessing disease status in patients who have undergone staging/cytoreductive surgery and primary chemotherapy. Traditionally, the operation is performed through a midline vertical incision as a „second-look laparotomy." Candidates for second-look surgery are patients who had advanced-stage disease at the time of diagnosis and have achieved an apparent clinical remission after their initial course of chemotherapy. The chances of finding persistent disease at the time of second look depends on multiple factors, such as FIGO stage and residual disease status after the primary surgery, but overall, approximately 50% of patients will have residual disease.

Shortly after Bagley and coworkers [22] published their results with „pretreatment peritoneoscopy," investigators at the NCI began reporting their experience with „second-look peritoneoscopy" [23]. Ozols et al. [24] updated the NCI experience with peritoneoscopy in the management of ovarian cancer in 1981. Sixty-six patients had second-look peritoneoscopies. Because of the laparoscopic detection of residual disease, 33 (50%) patients were spared unnecessary laparotomies. Twenty-two patients with negative peritoneoscopies underwent laparotomy, with residual ovarian cancer being found in 12 (55%). This 55% false-negative rate for peritoneoscopy when compared with laparotomy underscored the limitations of endoscopy at that time while emphasizing the need for subsequent laparotomy in patients who appeared disease-free at laparoscopy. However, the 50% reduction in the need for laparotomy illustrated one of the significant benefits of the minimally invasive approach.

Two recent studies have compared „modern" laparoscopy and laparotomy as second-look operations for patients with ovarian cancer. From our institution, Abu-Rustum et al. [25] compared the results of 31 second-look laparoscopies with 70 second-look laparotomies and found that laparoscopy was associated with less blood loss, less operative time, shorter hospital stay, and lower hospital charges per case (Table 1). All intraoperative and immediate postoperative complications were noted in patients who underwent laparotomy. The extent of surgery is similar for the laparoscopic procedure compared with an open laparotomy. Second-look laparoscopy frequently requires extensive adhesiolysis and lymphadenectomy. With a median follow-up of 22 months, recurrence after a negative second-look operation was 14% for both laparoscopy and laparotomy. Casey et al. [26] analyzed 121 second-look procedures with essentially identical results.

Second-look operations have contributed immeasurably to our understanding of the biologic behavior of ovarian cancer and to the development of effective chemotherapy for this disease. However, opponents of the procedure point out

Table 1. Comparison of second-look procedures (from [25] with permission)

Variable	Laparotomy (n=70)	Laparoscopy (n=31)	p
Operating room time (min)	153	129	<0.01
Estimated blood loss (ml)	208	27	<0.01
Hospital stay (days)	6.8	1.6	<0.01
Day of surgery charges (US $)	8,049	7,984	0.12
Total hospital charges (US $)	17,969	9,448	<0.01

that there is no objective evidence that it has a major impact on survival [27]. Despite this opposition, second-look surgery remains the gold standard in clinical protocols for determining the effectiveness of a specific treatment. Outside of clinical trials, second-look operations should only be undertaken if the anticipated findings will alter subsequent management [28]. At our institution, patients with either microscopic or no residual disease are given intraperitoneal chemotherapy after second-look surgery.

Cervical Neoplasms

According to FIGO conventions, cervical cancer is staged clinically, with the role of surgery in primary management reserved for the treatment of early-stage disease. These patients are often managed with a radical hysterectomy and bilateral pelvic lymphadenectomy. Patients who have more advanced-stage disease not amenable to resection are generally treated with radiation therapy, with or without chemotherapy. Over the past 10 years, numerous authors have investigated the use of laparoscopy in both the treatment of early-stage disease and the surgical staging of advanced disease.

Laparoscopy in the Treatment of Early-Stage Disease

Currently, there are two approaches to the endoscopic treatment of early-stage cervical cancer. The first approach combines laparoscopic lymphadenectomy, dissection of the uterine vessels, and division of the upper uterine attachments with a modified version of the Schauta radical vaginal hysterectomy. The second method involves almost the complete performance of a radical hysterectomy and bilateral pelvic lymphadenectomy laparoscopically. Although the two approaches differ in many aspects, what they do have in common is that they both must be considered experimental because neither method has been adequately studied and only a few surgeons in the world are fully qualified to perform either method.

Laparoscopically Assisted Radical Vaginal Hysterectomy

In 1987, Dargent [29] first described an endoscopic technique to remove pelvic lymph nodes in patients with early cervical cancer. He combined radical hysterectomy with the technique of „retroperitoneal pelviscopy" in 10 patients. Using this technique, Dargent was able to remove pelvic lymph nodes up to the bifurcation of the common iliac artery. Six patients underwent immediate laparotomy, and none had positive lymph nodes that were not identified laparoscopically.

Querleu and colleagues [30] subsequently described their transperitoneal laparoscopic approach to pelvic lymphadenectomy in early-stage cervical cancer. They performed laparoscopic pelvic lymph node dissections in 39 patients. The dissection was limited to the area below the common iliac vessels with a mean of 8.7 lymph nodes removed per patient. Thirty-two patients underwent a subsequent laparotomy with radical hysterectomy and removal of all remaining lymph node tissue. No residual lymph node metastases were found.

With the apparent efficacy of laparoscopic lymph node dissection and the familiarity of the transperitoneal approach, investigators have now begun combining laparoscopic lymphadenectomy with modifications of the Schauta radical vaginal hysterectomy as an alternative to traditional radical abdominal hysterectomy with pelvic lymphadenectomy for the treatment of early cervical cancer. Although different authors vary in what parts of the radical hysterectomy they perform endoscopically, not even those with extensive experience with the Schauta technique currently perform the whole radical hysterectomy vaginally [31].

To date, over 250 patients worldwide have undergone a laparoscopically assisted radical vaginal hysterectomy (LARVH) [32–38]. In 1993, Dargent and colleagues [33] presented not only one of the largest series of LARVH, but also the one with the longest follow-up. They performed 51 cases and reported a 3-year actuarial survival rate of 95.5% for patients with node-negative, stage IB and IIA disease. Furthermore, their average operating time was 93 min, with a reoperation and urinary tract fistula rate of 0%.

The more limited American experience with LARVH is somewhat different and reflects the fact that the majority of gynecologic oncologists in the United States have never performed a radical vaginal hysterectomy [34, 36]. In the largest American series, Hatch et al. [36] reported a mean operative time of 225 min. In the 37 cases, there were two bladder injuries, two ureterovaginal fistulas, and one large-bowel injury. Although LARVH appears feasible and its successful completion appears to reduce blood loss, decrease febrile morbidity, and shorten hospital stays when compared to traditional laparotomy, the reports by Hatch et al. and others highlight many of the substantial questions that remain regarding the safety and adequacy of the procedure [35–37]. In most modern series of radical hysterectomy, the urinary tract injury rate should not exceed 1%.

Perhaps one of the most ingenious applications of laparoscopic surgery in the management of early cervical cancer was first performed by Dargent in 1987 [39]. He combined laparoscopic pelvic lymphadenectomy with radical vaginal trachelectomy in women who desired to maintain their fertility. By retaining the body of the uterus, women preserved their reproductive function while theoretically receiving a satisfactory oncological procedure. Currently, the world literature is limited to 62 cases, but thus far, over a dozen healthy babies have been born from women who have undergone the procedure, with only four documented recurrences [40].

The Gynecologic Oncology Group (GOG) has recently closed a prospective clinical trial evaluating laparoscopic lymphadenectomy in women with early-stage cervical cancer. Seventy-three patients have been accrued who have undergone immediate laparotomy after transperitoneal laparoscopic pelvic and para-aortic lymph node sampling. The results and conclusions are not yet available. Although this GOG study will not be able to address any issues regarding the safety and efficacy of radical vaginal hysterectomy or radical vaginal trachelectomy, it may be the first step in answering some of the questions concerning the adequacy and adverse effects of laparoscopic lymphadenectomy in patients with early-stage cervical cancer.

Laparoscopic Radical Hysterectomy

Laparoscopic radical hysterectomy was first described by Canis et al. [41] and Nezhat et al. [42] in 1992. These early reports were questioned regarding the length of the procedure (8 and 7 h, respectively) and its radicality (10 and 14 pelvic nodes removed, respectively). More recent reports have demonstrated shorter operative times and higher lymph node yields [43–46].

Spirtos et al. [46] recently presented the largest series to date. With the use of argon beam coagulation and endoscopic staplers, 43 patients successfully underwent laparoscopic radical hysterectomy with aortic and pelvic lymphadenectomy. The average operating time was 225 min with an average blood loss of 250 ml. The mean number of removed lymph nodes was 32 (range 19–65). One patient developed a ureterovaginal fistula postoperatively requiring reoperation, and there has been one documented recurrence.

Although the English literature currently contains fewer than 100 cases of patients that have undergone laparoscopic radical hysterectomy, the technique offers many potential advantages over LARVH [41–46]. First, the majority of gynecologic oncologists in the United States are much more comfortable performing a traditional radical abdominal hysterectomy than a radical vaginal hysterectomy. Therefore, performance of a laparoscopic radical hysterectomy would require mastering the use of new surgical tools as opposed to learning an entirely new and rather difficult procedure [47]. Second, visualization of essential structures can be difficult during radical vaginal hysterectomy for even the most experienced vaginal surgeons. This problem should very rarely be the case during a laparoscopic radical hysterectomy. Finally, LARVH frequently requires perineal or vulvar incisions to facilitate the dissection. These incisions are avoided with the laparoscopic radical hysterectomy technique. Only time and future clinical trials will determine whether these potential advantages translate into improved patient outcomes.

▌ Laparoscopic Staging of Advanced-Stage Disease

Because the FIGO staging system for cervical cancer is a clinical one, the standard management for patients with advanced, unresectable disease does not include surgical evaluation. However, over 30% of cases of advanced disease will be inaccurately staged by clinical methods, and for this reason many investigators have studied the role of pretreatment surgical staging in these patients [48].

Based on its known patterns of spread, the pretreatment surgical staging of cervical cancer involves bilateral retroperitoneal lymph node assessment. The main proposed benefit of pretreatment staging is that it provides a more accurate definition of the extent of disease spread so that irradiation and/or chemotherapy can be better individualized. The disadvantages relate to the morbidity associated with a major surgical procedure that gives information that will benefit less than 10% of patients undergoing the operation [49]. Furthermore, a prolonged recovery period after pretreatment laparotomy can lead to significant delays in the initiation of definitive therapy.

Pretreatment surgical staging for patients with advanced cervical cancer remains a controversial issue. Adding to the controversy, many authors are now reporting the use of operative endoscopic techniques for pretreatment surgical staging. The purported advantages of the laparoscopic approach are the same delineation of the extent of disease as achieved with laparotomy but with less morbidity and essentially no delay in the initiation of definitive therapy.

One of the most significant problems with pretreatment laparotomy is the subsequent formation of intra-abdominal adhesions, which leads to a higher incidence of postirradiation enteric morbidity. Weiser et al. [50] have demonstrated that this morbidity can be reduced if the laparotomy and lymphadenectomy are performed via an extraperitoneal rather than a transperitoneal approach. Although clinical studies have not compared adhesion formation after extraperitoneal versus laparoscopic lymphadenectomy, animal studies have shown that adhesion formation is the same between the two [51–53].

In 1992, Childers and colleagues [54] reported on six patients with advanced cervical cancer who underwent preirradiation laparoscopic staging. All patients had clinical stage IIB disease or greater and negative lymph nodes on preoperative computed tomography (CT) scan. They all underwent pelvic and para-aortic lymph node sampling. Two patients were found to have positive pelvic nodes, one of which also had positive para-aortic nodes. These 6 patients were reported as part of a larger group of 18 patients with cervical cancer who underwent laparoscopic lymphadenectomy. The average number of lymph nodes removed laparoscopically for the whole group was 31.4, and there were no significant short-term complications.

Although studies such as the one by Childers et al. [54] have shown that laparoscopic pelvic lymphadenectomy is feasible and can be performed safely in patients with advanced cervical cancer, its clinical usefulness is questionable. Because these patients are generally going to receive whole-pelvic radiotherapy, the status of the pelvic lymph nodes will not have any impact on subsequent management. Therefore, most authors, including Childers and colleagues, are now sampling only the high pelvic and low para-aortic lymph nodes that lie outside the planned radiation field [38, 55–57]. If these lymph nodes are positive, then the radiation field can be extended to include the para-aortic nodes and/or chemotherapy can be given.

The largest experience with laparoscopic staging of advanced cervical cancer was recently reported by Chu et al. [38]. Twenty-eight patients with clinical stage IIB–IIIB cervical cancer underwent laparoscopic bilateral para-aortic lymph node dissections. An average of eight nodes were removed per patient, and the average operation time was 95 minutes. The one complication (3.6%) was bleeding from the inferior vena cava, which required laparotomy for correction. Ten patients (36%) had positive para-aortic nodes and were subsequently treated with extended-field radiation or chemotherapy with whole-pelvic irradiation. The patients with negative para-aortic nodes were given pelvic radiation alone. With a short mean follow-up of 18 months, only one patient has recurred.

Although this series by Chu et al. [38] again demonstrates the feasibility of laparoscopic lymphadenectomy and brings the total number of patients in the English literature with advanced disease who have undergone laparoscopic surgical staging to greater than 50, it also underscores the fact that studies with large patient numbers and long-term follow-up are lacking [55–57]. The GOG trial that is evaluating laparoscopic lymphadenectomy before planned laparotomy in women with early cervical cancer was originally proposed to also include laparoscopic staging for patients with advanced disease. However, the protocol was amended to investigate only the early-stage patients. Therefore, it is unlikely that the questions regarding the safety of preirradiation laparoscopic staging will be answered any time in the foreseeable future [47]. Currently, we use this approach to pretreatment staging on a limited basis at our institution.

Endometrial Neoplasms

The majority of women with endometrial cancer present with disease apparently confined to the uterus. Surgical removal of the uterus is the most important step in the treatment of these patients with clinical stage I disease. However, studies done by the GOG have demonstrated that over 20% of patients with endometrial cancer clinically confined to the uterus will be found to have disease outside the uterus at staging laparotomy [58]. Therefore, in 1988, FIGO recommended that the staging of endometrial cancer be changed from a clinical to a surgical system [59]. The surgical staging procedure includes peritoneal washings, removal of the uterus and adnexae, and retroperitoneal lymph node sampling. Although most of the original reports of laparoscopic lymph node dissection involved patients with cervical cancer, its application may be the most feasible and useful for women with apparent early-stage endometrial cancer.

Laparoscopically Assisted Surgical Staging

By combining operative laparoscopy with vaginal hysterectomy, laparoscopically assisted surgical staging (LASS) has been proposed as an alternative to laparotomy for patients with early endometrial cancer. Operative laparoscopy allows for the assessment of the intraperitoneal cavity, the ability to obtain peritoneal washings, and the guaranteed removal of the ovaries. Most importantly, lymph node sampling can also be performed laparoscopically in indicated cases (varies depending on the institution, but generally those cases with high-grade tumors and/or tumor invasion to the outer half of the myometrium). The uterus and cervix are removed during the vaginal portion of the procedure as in a laparoscopically assisted vaginal hysterectomy (LAVH) for benign disease [60].

The first series of LASS procedures for endometrial cancer was reported by Childers et al. [61] in 1993. Fifty-nine patients with clinical stage I endometrial carcinoma underwent laparoscopic evaluation. Six patients were found to have intraperitoneal disease and did not undergo further laparoscopic staging. Of the remaining 53 patients, 52 underwent an LAVH and 29 were considered candidates for laparoscopic lymph node sampling. The lymphadenectomy was performed successfully by laparoscopy in 93% of these patients, although bilateral para-aortic lymph node sampling was not achieved in all. The estimated blood loss was less than 200 ml, and the average hospital stay was 2.9 days. There were two significant complications: a transected ureter and a cystotomy, which both required repair via laparotomy. Although this study demonstrated the feasibility of the LASS procedure and identified obesity as a limiting factor, the number of lymph nodes removed laparoscopically, the comparative costs of the procedure, and long-term follow-up were not discussed.

Many of these issues have been recently addressed. From our institution, Gemignani et al. [62] compared the clinical outcomes and hospital charges for 320 patients with endometrial cancer treated by laparoscopically assisted vaginal hysterectomy (LAVH), adnexectomy versus traditional laparotomy, complete hysterectomy, and adnexectomy (TAH). The patients managed laparoscopically had

Table 2. Operative data and charges (from [62] with permission)

Variable	LAVH	TAH	p Value
Lymph node sampling (%)	11/69 (16)	113/251 (45)	$p<0.01$
Mean pathological lymph node yield	7 nodes	6 nodes	NS
Range	(0–14 nodes)	(0–30 nodes)	
OR time	214.6 min	144.5 min	$p<0.05$
Estimated blood loss	219 cc	215 cc	NS
Length of stay (median)	2 days	6 days	$p<0.05$
Nodal sampling group	2 days	6 days	
No nodal sampling group	2 days	6 days	
Total charges	US $11,826	US $15,189	$p<0.05$
Nodal sampling group	US $11,790	US $15,220	
No nodal sampling group	US $12,680	US $15,150	
OR charges	US $4,095	US $3,239	$p<0.05$
OR supply charges	US $1,618	US $83	$p<0.05$
Room charges	US $3,130	US $6,960	$p<0.05$

Fig. 1. Survival analysis. Follow-up data available for 65 LAVH patients and 235 TAH patients. There is no significant difference in disease recurrence between the two groups. (Used with permission from [62])

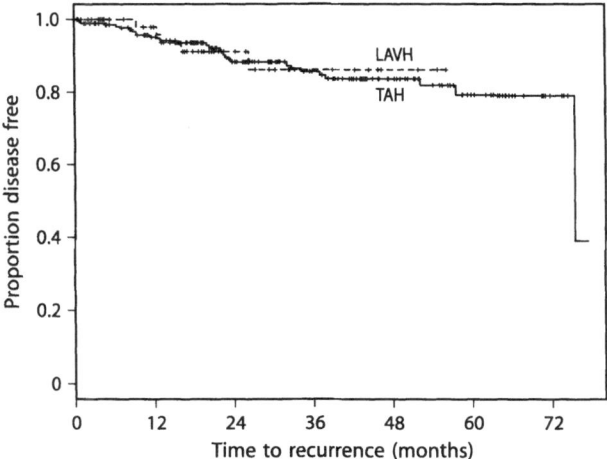

significantly fewer complications, shorter hospitalizations, and lower overall hospital charges than those who underwent laparotomy (Table 2). Furthermore, there was no statistically significant difference in the recurrence rates between the two groups (4.5% with a mean follow-up of 12.4 months for the laparoscopy group versus 13.9% with a mean follow-up of 24 months for the laparotomy group) (Fig. 1). Approximately one-third to one-half of all patients with endometrial cancer treated at our institution are considered candidates for a laparos--copically assisted procedure.

The safety, efficacy, and cost savings of LASS are currently being evaluated in a prospective manner. The GOG is performing a randomized Phase III trial designed to compare the differences between LASS versus staging via laparotomy in the management of women with early endometrial cancer. Variables that will be assessed include adequacy of staging, complications, operative time, hospital stay, total procedural costs, and quality of life. To date, 91 patients have been entered in the trial and accrual is still ongoing.

Complications

Although the complexity of the laparoscopic procedures performed over the past 10 years has increased, so has the number of complications. Data regarding gynecologic laparoscopic complications are now beginning to accumulate [63, 64]. However, because of the relatively short interval during which operative laparoscopic techniques have been applied in the management of gynecologic cancer, there are very few data on the complication rates in this setting [65].

Abu-Rustum et al. [66] recently compared the complication rates of laparoscopic gynecologic procedures for 410 patients with malignant disease versus 312 patients with benign conditions. The three most common procedures were bilateral salpingo-oophorectomy, laparoscopically assisted vaginal hysterectomy, and second-look laparoscopy. Although the procedures undertaken were generally more complex in the patients with malignancy (e.g., retroperitoneal lymph nodes were never sampled in patients with benign disease), the complication rates were not statistically different (4.8% for patients with benign conditions versus 8.3% for patients with malignant disease). For the 410 patients with malignancy, the most common complications were wound infection, incidental enterotomy, incidental cystotomy, and abdominal wall hematoma. The incidence of each of these complications was between 1.0% and 1.5%. The authors emphasized that the use of an open technique during initial peritoneal access is responsible for the absence of major vessel injury and the low enterotomy rate (0.4%) at initial trocar insertion for the 722 total cases. In a series of 90 open laparoscopies performed in 89 oncological patients, Decloedt et al. [67] came to a similar conclusion regarding the open versus the closed technique.

Cutaneous trocar site metastases have been reported in patients with cervical, endometrial, and ovarian cancer [68–70]. The majority of patients who have developed these metastases have ovarian cancer. Kruitwagen et al. [71] recently reported that 7 of 43 patients (16%) who had undergone laparoscopy before ovarian cancer debulking developed trocar site metastases. This contrasts with the 1.1% rate described in 88 patients with intraperitoneal cancer (70 of whom had ovarian cancer) previously described by Childers and colleagues [72]. Although the actual rate of trocar site metastasis in patients with gynecologic malignancies is yet to be defined, it appears most likely that the frequency will vary depending on the type of malignancy and the volume of the disease.

Other reported but rare complications unique to the use of operative laparoscopy in the management of gynecologic cancer include major vessel injury during retroperitoneal lymph node sampling and pelvic nerve injury during laparoscopic lymphadenectomy [65].

▌ Conclusion

Laparoscopic surgery has been successfully applied to the management of gynecologic cancers at our institution over the past 6 years. Currently, 25% of all surgical cases performed by the Gynecology Service include a laparoscopic component. The primary use of laparoscopy has been in the management of known or suspected ovarian neoplasms and in the management of endometrial cancer. It is likely that future developments will continue to expand the indications for laparoscopy. However, surgeons must continue to carefully analyze the clinical and economic outcomes, to ensure that we continue to offer our patients the optimal and most cost-effective therapy available.

References

1. Landis SH, Murray T, Bolden S, Wingo PA (1999) Cancer statistics, 1999. CA Cancer J Clin 49:8–31
2. Velebil P, Wingo PA, Xia Z, Wilcox LS, Peterson HB (1995) Rate of hospitalization for gyne-cologic disorders among reproductive-age women in the United States. Obstet Gynecol 86:764–769
3. Bast RC Jr, Klug TL, St John E, Jenison E, Niloff JM, Lazarus H, Berkowitz RS, Leavitt T, Griffiths CT, Parker L, Zurawski VR Jr, Knapp RC (1983) A radioimmunoassay using a mon-oclonal antibody to monitor the course of epithelial ovarian cancer. N Engl J Med 309:883–887
4. Malkasian GD Jr, Knapp RC, Lavin PT, Zurawski VR Jr, Podratz KC (1988) Preoperative eval-uation of serum CA 125 levels in premenopausal and postmenopausal patients with pelvic masses: discrimination of benign from malignant disease. Am J Obstet Gynecol 159:341–346
5. Vasilev SA, Schlaerth JB, Campeau J, Morrow CP (1988) Serum CA 125 levels in preoperative evaluation of pelvic masses. Obstet Gynecol 71:751–756
6. Finkler NJ, Benacerraf B, Lavin PT, Wojciechowski C, Knapp RC (1988) Comparison of serum CA 125, clinical impression, and ultrasound in the preoperative evaluation of ovari-an masses. Obstet Gynecol 72:659–664
7. Granberg S, Wikland M, Jansson I (1989) Macroscopic characterization of ovarian tumors and the relation to the histological diagnosis: Criteria to be used for ultrasound evaluation. Gynecol Oncol 35:139–144
8. Lerner JP, Timor-Tritsch IE, Federman A, Abramovich G (1994) Transvaginal ultrasono-graphic characterization of ovarian masses with an improved, weighted scoring system. Am J Obstet Gynecol 170:81–85
9. Fleischer AC, Cullinan JA, Kepple DM, Williams LL (1993) Conventional and color Doppler transvaginal sonography of pelvic masses: a comparison of relative histologic specificities. J Ultrasound Med 12:705–712
10. Flynn M, Niloff JM (1995) Minilaparotomy for the ambulatory management of ovarian cysts. Am J Obstet Gynecol 173:1727–1730
11. Pittaway DE, Takacs P, Bauguess P (1994) Laparoscopic adnexectomy: A comparison with laparotomy. Am J Obstet Gynecol 171:385–391
12. Canis M, Mage G, Pouly JL, Wattiez A, Manhes H, Bruhat MA (1994) Laparoscopic diagnosis of adnexal cystic masses: a 12-year experience with long-term follow-up. Obstet Gynecol 83:707–712
13. Nezhat F, Nezhat C, Welander CE, Benigno B (1992) Four ovarian cancers diagnosed during laparoscopic management of 1011 women with adnexal masses. Am J Obstet Gynecol 167:790–796
14. Mecke H, Lehmann-Willenbrock E, Ibrahim M, Semm K (1992) Pelviscopic treatment of ovarian cysts in premenopausal women. Gynecol Obstet Invest 34:36–42
15. Robinson WR, Curtin JP, Morrow CP (1992) Operative staging and conservative surgery in the management of low malignant potential ovarian tumors. Int J Gynecol Cancer 2:113–118
16. Menzin AW, Rubin SC, Noumoff JS, LiVolsi VA (1995) The accuracy of a frozen section diag-nosis of borderline ovarian malignancy. Gynecol Oncol 59:183–185
17. Webb MJ, Decker DG, Mussey E, Williams TJ (1973) Factor influencing survival in stage I ovarian cancer. Am J Obstet Gynecol 116:222–228
18. Dembo AJ, Davy M, Stenwig AE, Berle EJ, Bush RS, Kjorstad K (1990) Prognostic factors in patients with stage I epithelial ovarian cancer. Obstet Gynecol 75:263–273

19. Parker WH, Levine RL, Howard FM, Sansone B, Berek JS (1994) A multicenter study of laparoscopic management of selected cystic adnexal masses in postmenopausal women. J Am Coll Surg 179:733–737

20. Childers JM, Lang J, Surwit EA, Hatch KD (1995) Laparoscopic surgical staging of ovarian cancer. Gynecol Oncol 59:25–35

21. Chi DS, Curtin JP, Barakat RR (1995) Laparoscopic management of adnexal masses in women with a history of nongynecologic malignancy. Obstet Gynecol 86: 964–8

22. Bagley CM Jr, Young RC, Schein PS, Chabner BA, DeVita VT (1973) Ovarian carcinoma metastatic to the diaphragm-frequently undiagnosed at laparotomy. A Preliminary Report. Am J Obstet Gynecol 116:397–400

23. Rosenoff SH, DeVita T Jr, Hubbard S, Young RC (1975) Peritoneoscopy in the staging and follow-up of ovarian cancer. Semin Oncol 2:223–228

24. Ozols RF, Fisher RI, Anderson T, Makuch R, Young RC (1981) Peritoneoscopy in the management of ovarian cancer. Am J Obstet Gynecol 140:611–619

25. Abu-Rustum NR, Barakat RR, Siegel PL, Venkatraman E, Curtin JP, Hoskins WJ (1996) Second-look operation for epithelial ovarian cancer: laparoscopy or laparotomy? Obstet Gynecol 88:549–543

26. Casey AC, Farias-Eisner R, Pisani AL, Cirisano FD, Kim YB, Muderspach L, Futoran R, Leuchter RS, Lagasse LD, Karlan BY (1996) What is the role of reassessment laparoscopy in the management of gynecologic cancers in 1995? Gynecol Oncol 60:454–461

27. Creasman WT (1994) Second-look laparotomy in ovarian cancer. Gynecol Oncol 55:S122–S127

28. National Institutes of Health Consensus Development Conference Statement (1994) Ovarian cancer: screening, treatment, and follow-up. Gynecol Oncol 55:S4–S14

29. Dargent D (1987) A new future for Schauta's operation through pre-surgical retroperitoneal pelviscopy? Eur J Gynaecol Oncol 8:292

30. Querleu D, Leblanc E, Castelain B (1991) Laparoscopic pelvic lymphadenectomy in the staging of early carcinoma of the cervix. Am J Obstet Gynecol 164:579–581

31. Dargent D (1993) Laparoscopic surgery and gynecologic cancer. Curr Opin Obstet Gynecol 5:294–300

32. Querleu D (1993) Laparoscopically assisted radical vaginal hysterectomy. Gynecol Oncol 51:248–254

33. Dargent D, Mathevet P (1995) Schauta's vaginal hysterectomy combined with laparoscopic lymphadenectomy. Baillieres Clin Obstet Gynaecol 9:691–705

34. Kadar N (1994) Laparoscopic vaginal radical hysterectomy: an operative technique and its evolution. Gynaecol Endoscopy 3:109

35. Roy M, Plante M, Renaud MC, Tetu B (1996) Vaginal radical hysterectomy versus abdominal radical hysterectomy in the treatment of early-stage cervical cancer. Gynecol Oncol 62(3):336–339

36. Hatch KD, Hallum AV 3rd, Nour M (1996) New surgical approaches to treatment of cervical cancer. J Natl Cancer Inst Monogr 21:71–75

37. Possover M, Krause N, Schneider A (1998) Identification of the ureter and dissection of the bladder pillar in laparoscopic-assisted radical vaginal hysterectomy. Obstet Gynecol 91:139–143

38. Chu KK, Chang SD, Chen FP, Soong YK (1997) Laparoscopic surgical staging in cervical cancer – preliminary experience among Chinese. Gynecol Oncol 64(1):49–53

39. Roy M, Plante M (1998) Pregnancies after radical vaginal trachelectomy for early-stage cervical cancer. Am J Obstet Gynecol 179:1491–1496

40. Plante M, Roy M (1997) Radical Trachelectomy. Operat Tech Gynecol Surg 2:187

41. Canis M, Mage G, Wattiez A (1992) Vaginally assisted laparoscopic radical hysterectomy. J Gynecol Surg 8:103
42. Nezhat CR, Burrell MO, Nezhat FR, Benigno BB, Welander CE (1992) Laparoscopic radical hysterectomy with paraaortic and pelvic node dissection. Am J Obstet Gynecol 166(3):864–865
43. Nezhat CR, Nezhat FR, Burrell MO, Ramirez CE, Welander C, Carrodeguas J, Nezhat CH (1993) Laparoscopic radical hysterectomy and laparoscopic-assisted vaginal radical hysterectomy with pelvic and para-aortic lymph node dissection. J Gynecol Surg 9:105–120
44. Sedlacek TV (1995) Laparoscopic radical hysterectomy: the next evolutionary step in the treatment of invasive cervical cancer. J Gynecol Tech 1:223
45. Spirtos NM, Schlaerth JB, Kimball RE, Leiphart VM, Ballon SC (1996) Laparoscopic radical hysterectomy (type III) with aortic and pelvic lymphadenectomy. Am J Obstet Gynecol 174(6):1763–1767
46. Spirtos NM, Ballon SC, Perez GM, Stern JL, Schlaerth JB (1998) Laparoscopic radical hysterectomy (type III) with aortic and pelvic lymphadenectomy: surgical morbidity and short-term follow-up. Gynecol Oncol 68:106
47. Montz FJ, Schlaerth JB (1995) Laparoscopic surgery: does it have a role in the management of gynecologic malignancies? Clin Obstet Gynecol 38(2):426–435
48. Morrow CP, Curtin JP, Townsend DE (1993) Tumors of the cervix. In: Synopsis of gynecologic oncology. Churchill Livingstone Inc., New York
49. Potish RA, Twiggs LB, Okagaki T, Prem KA, Adcock LL (1985) Therapeutic implications of the natural history of advanced cervical cancer as defined by pretreatment surgical staging. Cancer 56:956–960
50. Weiser EB, Bundy BN, Hoskins WJ, Heller PB, Whittington RR, DiSaia PJ, Curry SL, Schlaerth J, Thigpen JT (1989) Extraperitoneal versus transperitoneal selective paraaortic lymphadenectomy in the pretreatment surgical staging of advanced cervical carcinoma (a Gynecologic Oncology Group study). Gynecol Oncol 33:283–289
51. Fowler JM, Hartenbach EM, Reynolds HT, Borner J, Carter JR, Carlson JW, Twiggs LB, Carson LF (1994) Pelvic adhesion formation after pelvic lymphadenectomy: comparison between transperitoneal laparoscopy and extraperitoneal laparotomy in a porcine model. Gynecol Oncol 55:25–28
52. Lanvin D, Elhage A, Henry B, Leblanc E, Querleu D, Delobelle-Deroide A (1997) Accuracy and safety of laparoscopic lymphadenectomy: an experimental prospective randomized study. Gynecol Oncol 67:83–87
53. Chen MD, Teigen GA, Reynolds HT, Johnson PR, Fowler JM (1998) Laparoscopy versus laparotomy: an evaluation of adhesion formation after pelvic and paraaortic lymphadenectomy in a porcine model. Am J Obstet Gynecol 178:499–503
54. Childers JM, Hatch K, Surwit EA (1992) The role of laparoscopic lymphadenectomy in the management of cervical carcinoma. Gynecol Oncol 47:38–43
55. Childers JM, Hatch KD, Tran AN, Surwit EA (1993) Laparoscopic para-aortic lymphadenectomy in gynecologic malignancies. Obstet Gynecol 82:741–747
56. Kadar N, Pelosi MA (1994) Can cervical cancer be adequately staged by laparoscopic aortic lymphadenectomy? Gynaecol Endoscopy 3:213
57. Su TH, Wang KG, Yang YC, Hong BK, Huang SH (1995) Laparoscopic para-aortic lymph node sampling in the staging of invasive cervical carcinoma: including a comparative study of 21 laparotomy cases. Int J Gynaecol Obstet 49:311–318
58. Creasman WT, Morrow CP, Bundy BN, Homesley HD, Graham JE, Heller PB (1987) Surgical pathologic spread patterns of endometrial cancer: a Gynecologic Oncology Group study. Cancer 60 [Suppl 8]:2035–2041

59. International Federation of Gynecology and Obstetrics: annual report on the treatment of gynecologic cancer (1989) Int J Gynecol Obstet 28:189
60. Morrow CP, Curtin JP (1996) Minimal access surgery. In: Gynecologic cancer surgery. Churchill Livingstone Inc, New York
61. Childers JM, Brzechffa PR, Hatch KD, Surwit EA (1993) Laparoscopically assisted surgical staging (LASS) of endometrial cancer. Gynecol Oncol 51:33–38
62. Gemignani ML, Curtin JP, Zelmanovich J, Patel DA, Venkatraman E, Barakat RR (1999) Laparoscopic-assisted vaginal hysterectomy for endometrial cancer: clinical outcomes and hospital charges. Gynecol Oncol 73:5–11
63. Siren PH, Kurki T (1997) A nationwide analysis of laparoscopic complications. Obstet Gynecol 89:108
64. Jansen FW, Kapiteyn K, Trimbos-Kemper T, Hermans J, Trimbos JB (1997) Complications of laparoscopy: a prospective multicentre observational study. Br J Obstet Gynaecol 104:595–600
65. Montz FJ (1997) Complications of gynecologic oncology laparoscopic surgery. Operative Techniques in Gynecologic Surgery 2:219
66. Abu-Rustum N, Barakat RR, Curtin JP (1999) Laparoscopic complications in gynecologic surgery for benign or malignant disease. Gynecol Oncol
67. Decloedt J, Berteloot P, Vergote I (1997) The feasibility of open laparoscopy in gynecologic-oncologic patients. Gynecol Oncol 66:138–140
68. Naumann RW, Spencer S (1997) Case report: an umbilical metastasis after laparoscopy for squamous cell carcinoma of the cervix . Gynecol Oncol 64:507–509
69. Wang PH, Yen MS, Yuan CC, Chao KC, Ng HT, Lee WL, Chao HT (1997) Case report: Port site metastasis after laparoscopic-assisted vaginal hysterectomy for endometrial cancer: possible mechanisms and prevention. Gynecol Oncol 66:151–155
70. Gleeson NC, Nicosia SV, Mark JE, Hoffman MS, Cavanagh D (1993) Abdominal wall metastases from ovarian cancer after laparoscopy. Am J Obstet Gynecol 169:522–523
71. Kruitwagen RF, Swinkels BM, Keyser KG, Doesburg WH, Schijf CP (1996) Incidence and effect on survival of abdominal wall metastases at trocar or puncture sites following laparoscopy or paracentesis in women with ovarian cancer. Gynecol Oncol 60:233–237
72. Childers JM, Aqua KA, Surwit EA, Hallum AV, Hatch KD (1994) Abdominal-wall tumor implantation after for malignant conditions. Obstet Gynecol 84:765–769

Indications in Urologic Tumors

P. Russo

Laparoscopy in Urologic Oncology

Introduction

Over the last 8 years, there has been a marked expansion in urologic laparoscopic techniques from simple diagnostic procedures to complex ablative and reconstructive operations done in specialized medical centers with committed clinical and research personnel [1]. In urologic oncology today, laparoscopy remains a valid tool for use in precise indications but it has not achieved widespread application because of limitations defined by the diseases at hand as well as the available technology. Although the surgical literature has reports of laparoscopy being applied to the wide range of genitourinary cancers (e.g., laparoscopic nephrectomy, laparoscopic nephroureterectomy, laparoscopic retroperitoneal lymph node dissection), our center as well as others has yet to embrace some procedures because of concerns regarding the thoroughness of the operations, the possibility of tumor spillage and port site contamination, and difficulties in retrieving the specimens from the abdominal cavity. In addition, because of the practical concerns regarding the steep learning curves required to gain expertise in these more complicated procedures, as well the costs of additional operating room time in what otherwise are straightforward operations, there has been a notable decrease in enthusiasm for the very complex laparoscopic procedures. In this chapter, I will review the principal features of laparoscopy in urologic oncology with an emphasis on its current role in the management of cancers encountered at Memorial Sloan-Kettering Cancer Center (MSKCC).

Laparoscopy and Prostate Cancer

The principal laparoscopic urologic procedure at MSKCC is laparoscopic pelvic lymph node dissection (LPLND). The finding of a regional metastasis from prostate cancer to pelvic (obturator fossa) lymph nodes is indicative of systemic disease and uniformly predicts the failure of local treatments such as radical surgery or radiation therapy to achieve a cure [2, 3]. Historically, open bilateral pelvic lymph node dissection, either as a separate staging procedure before external beam irradiation, interstitial radioactive iodine implantation, or perineal radical prostatectomy, or when combined with radical retropubic prostatectomy, was the definitive means of assessing the regional nodes. For most urologic oncologists, the finding of metastatic lymph nodes by frozen or permanent section would prompt the termination of the definitive local treatment procedure in an attempt to avoid unpleasant local side effects of treatment without the hope for cure. Improvements in the noninvasive imaging techniques of MRI and CT scanning now allow for detection of bulky regional nodal involvement with tissue diagnostic confirmation then obtained by CT-guided percutaneous biopsy or aspiration cytology [4]. Such patients can readily be excluded from more invasive diagnostic procedures to determine the nodal status. However, microscopic nodal spread cannot be detected by CT or MRI [5].

On its inception in the early 1990s, laparoscopic lymphadenectomy provided the introduction of adult urology to the already established field of laparoscopy [6]. Today, laparoscopic lymphadenectomy is the laparoscopic procedure most commonly performed in adult urology. The evolution of laparoscopic lymph node dissection techniques occurred during the transition between the era of the clinical diagnosis of prostate cancer to the current serological diagnosis of prostate cancer [7]. Within this time frame, reports from a number of investigators confirmed that the laparoscopic procedure was safe, the yield of lymph nodes was comparable to that of the open node dissection, the need for extended analgesics was reduced, and postoperative recovery with return to normal daily activities was dramatically improved [8–10].

The evolution of the serological diagnosis of prostate cancer over the last 10 years by the widespread application of prostate-specific antigen (PSA) [11] and the free-to-total PSA ratio [12] coupled with ready access to transrectal ultrasound-guided needle biopsy of the prostate [13] has created a marked migration in prostate cancer to an earlier stage at the time of diagnosis. Instead of patients presenting with locally advanced, symptomatic tumors (T2C, T3), most patients now have cancers detected in normal-feeling prostate glands (T1C) in evaluations initiated by an elevated serum PSA or free-to-total PSA ratio of less than 18%. During this time frame, the overall yearly incidence in prostate cancer in the United States jumped from 80,000 to a high of more than 300,000 and down to the current level of 200,000 new cases. With clinicians now able to carefully select patients for treatment from the large pool of serologically detected patients, many with normal-appearing pelvic CT or MRI scans, the rate of positive pelvic lymph nodes at presentation has decreased from 30%–40% to the 5% range [14]. Thus the need to obtain pathological assessment of the regional nodes before definitive treatment in all cases has substantially diminished in importance [15]. In addition, clinical investigators have constructed normograms predictive of pathological outcomes based on preoperative PSA, a pathological Gleason score, and clinical stage, further defining the ideal surgical candidate [16, 17]. These same parameters were also effective in predicting the likelihood of a nodal metastasis in patients presenting with prostate cancer [18, 19].

At MSKCC we have incorporated LPLND as a means of assessing regional nodes only in poor prognostic patients or patients with suspicious nodes on a pelvic imaging study. Patients with clinical factors associated with an increased risk for nodal metastases, including any one of the following alone or in combination, are candidates for LPLND: (a) PSA >20 ng/ml, (b) Gleason histological

Table 1. Current indications for laparoscopic lymph node dissection at MSKCC

PSA >20 ng/ml
Gleason histological score >7
Serum acid phosphatase elevation
Locally advanced tumor

score >7, (c) serum acid phosphatase elevation, (d) locally advanced tumor (T3) (Table 1).

Between June 1993 and July1996, 24 patients with a PSA concentration of more than 20 ng/ml (n=19, 79%), elevation of serum acid phosphatase (n=4, 17%), and digital rectal exams consistent with T3 lesions (n=14, 58%) underwent pretreatment LPLND. Six patients (25%) had metastatic lymph nodes detected. Five of the six patients had palpable T3 (A–C) lesions, thus confirming the high-risk nature of the selected patients. In this series, an average of 10.8 lymph nodes were removed during a mean operating time of 174 min. As in other reported series of LPLND, there were no conversions to open laparotomy, blood loss was minimal, there was an early resumption of oral intake, and analgesic requirements were minimal. The average postoperative hospitalization was 1.2 days [20]. Perioperative complications were limited to two patients sustaining lacerations to branches of the inferior epigastric vessels handled by suture ligation of the trocar sites.

At the present time at MSKCC, LPLND is reserved for the above-described poor prognostic patient who has clinically localized disease with a PSA of more than 20 ng/ml, T3 lesion, a high-grade cancer, a negative pelvic CT or MRI, in whom curative local treatment is being contemplated. A positive seminal vesicle biopsy has also been identified as a poor prognostic indicator of pelvic nodal metastases [21, 22]. In addition, poor prognostic patients entered in high-risk protocols combining androgen ablation, systemic chemotherapy, and, if clinical response is good, curative consolidation therapy with radical prostatectomy or external beam irradiation therapy may be assessed with LPLND if equivocal nodes are observed on pretreatment imaging. This role for LPLND is now widely accepted in urologic oncology.

Laparoscopic Node Dissection: Applications in Other Malignancies

The experience acquired in learning LPLND has been applied to selected cases of poor prognostic invasive bladder cancer, penile cancer, and urethral cancer to confirm the presence of regional metastatic disease in which CT-guided biopsy is not possible [23]. The usual setting is that of an advanced unresectable primary tumor with confirmation of the extent of metastatic disease assisting the consulting oncologists in selecting the appropriate systemic chemotherapy regimen for the patient. This having been done, the goal of systemic chemotherapy is to significantly downstage the patient to the point of resectability [24]. These same laparoscopic techniques are also being applied by our colleagues for staging in cases of pelvic metastatic melanoma and cervical carcinoma. After neoadjuvant chemotherapy and before definitive laparotomy with resection, diagnostic laparoscopy has been performed to rule out peritoneal metastatic disease as well as to assist in the diagnosis of malignant retroperitoneal fibrosis [25].

Testicular Cancer

Reports exist in the literature concerning laparoscopic retroperitoneal lymph node dissection (RPLND) for patients with I nonseminomatous germ cell tumors (NSGCT) [26]. This procedure has been performed at a limited number of centers around the world and has been described, even by surgeons with considerable expertise, as a very demanding and time-consuming procedure [27]. Operative time in the initial experience (<100 reported laparoscopic RPLNDs) has been long (3.5–8 h) with difficulties in gaining access to the retro-aortic, and retrocaval lymph nodes reported. This raises the possibility that laparoscopic RPLND may be more of a node sampling than a true dissection [28, 29]. Current strategies to preserve sympathetic nerves allowing for antegrade ejaculation have not been similarly described in laparoscopic RPLND and may not be technically possible with the current instrumentation. For patients with clinical stage I NSGCT (tumor markers returned to normal by half-life, negative abdominal/pelvic CT, normal chest X-ray, no vascular or lymphatic invasion in the primary tumor), the options of a careful surveillance-only approach after radical orchiectomy (20% relapse rate in the absence of lymphatic or vascular invasion in the primary tumor within 2 years) vs. bilateral nerve-sparing open RPLND (with 90% preservation of antegrade ejaculation) are available. Despite the technical advances described in the literature, data do not currently exist in numbers with sufficient follow-up to confirm that laparoscopic RPLND is comparable to the open technique. Whether laparoscopic RPLND (node sampling of the primary landing zones) can be validated as an alternative approach in centers that combine adequate laparoscopic expertise with sufficient numbers of patients with testicular cancer remains to be seen. To date, MSKCC has not made laparoscopic RPLND an integral part of the management approach to stage I NSGCT. To my knowledge, there are no reports of postchemotherapy laparoscopic RPLND in the world's literature. It is doubtful that a complete and thorough dissection after chemotherapy, which is often complicated by dense adherence of residual disease or teratoma to the great vessels, can adequately be approached by laparoscopy in a safe, thorough, and timely fashion.

At MSKCC, we have reserved laparoscopy in testicular tumors to the search for the impalpable, cryptorchid testis with intra-abdominal location [30, 31] as well as the identification and resection of intra-abdominal testicular tumors [32, 33]. We await further reports concerning the efficacy of laparoscopic RPLND.

Laparoscopy and the Kidney

Because of the efforts of committed investigators, laparoscopic techniques have evolved, allowing for five-port transperitoneal resection of kidneys for both benign and malignant disease as well as for donor nephrectomy [34, 35, 36]. As in many laparoscopic procedures, the dividends of reduced hospital stay, reduced analgesic requirements in the postoperative period, and a faster return to normal activities and work were offset by a lengthy operating time, double that of the open nephrectomies. In addition, delivering the surgical specimen by organ entrapment techniques and tissue morcellation has led to concerns about seeding the peritoneal cavity or port sites with tumor cells as well as inaccuracies in pathological assessment. Investigators have recently utilized a 6.5-cm suprapubic incision to deliver the specimen intact in an attempt to address some of these concerns [37]. In the initial combined American laparoscopic nephrectomy experience of 185 cases, complications occurred in 12% of patients with benign diseases of the kidney and in 34% of those patients with renal cancer. Intraoperative complications related to vascular injury, splenic injury, and pneumothorax led to open surgical intervention in 8 of 185 cases [38].

Tumors most amenable to laparoscopic resection (P1, P2) are now being aggressively approached by partial nephrectomy in the strategy known as „nephron-sparing" surgery, which, to date, provides local control and cure rates similar to those of radical nephrectomy with a low expected rate (1%–3%) of local recurrence (new tumor formation) in the operated kidney [39–41]. Laparoscopic surgeons have been applying added instrumentation such as intraoperative ultrasound, the laparoscopic tourniquet, and the argon beam coagulator to initiate an experience with laparoscopic partial nephrectomy for both benign and malignant lesions [42, 43]. In these laparoscopic partial nephrectomies the operating team, through separate ports, uses the tourniquet to hold and compress the designated site of renal incision and the argon beam to compress and coagulate the cut renal surface. Currently, long-term reports detailing late complications and tumor control rates are anticipated.

Reports have appeared in the literature describing a procedure for laparoscopically assisted nephrectomy, which makes use of an abdominal incision to assist in the mobilization and removal of the specimen. This approach seemed to substantially shorten the operating time while still allowing for the rapid recovery found in the totally laparoscopic procedure [44, 45]. Laparoscopically assisted abdominal surgery has definitely gained a place in the operative approach to gynecologic and colorectal tumors and may play a role in the future in the management of renal tumors.

Santiago and colleagues recently reported the use of laparoscopically assisted renal cyst aspiration in patients with complex renal cysts. After the cyst fluid was sent for immediate cytology, 5 of 31 patients (14%) were found to have cystic renal cell carcinoma and then went on to have a radical or partial nephrectomy performed [46].

Despite the innovative clinical research techniques involving laparoscopic renal surgery described above, to date the Urologic Service at MSKCC has not embraced these techniques. It is clear from the literature that laparoscopic renal surgery is more difficult than LPLND and the more routine diagnostic procedures. Even in the hands of clinical investigators whose major interest is laparoscopy, the procedures are long, often complicated, and subject to a very steep learning curve. Institutions such as ours, where operating room time is in great demand, await the long-term results of this initial experience, as well as the technical improvements that may make laparoscopic renal surgery more widely appealing.

References

1. Gill IS, Clayman RV, McDougall E (1995) Advances in urologic laparoscopy. J Urol 154:1275–1294
2. Steinberg GD, Epstein JI, Piantadosi S, Walsh PC (1990) Management of stage D1 adenocarcinoma of the prostate. The Johns Hopkins experience 1874–1987. J Urol 144:1425–1432
3. Gervasi LA, Mata J, Easley JD, Wilbanks JH, Seale-Hawkins C, Carlton E, Scardino PT (1989) Prognostic significance of lymph node metastases in prostate cancer. J Urol 142:332–336
4. van Poppel H, Ameye F, Oyen R, van de Voorde W, Baerrt L (1994) Accuracy of combined computerized tomography and fine needle aspiration cytology in lymph node staging of localized prostatic carcinoma. Urol 151:1310–1314
5. Hricak H, Dooms GC, Jeffery RB (1987) Prostatic carcinoma: staging by clinical assessment, CT, and MR imaging. Radiology 162:331–336
6. Schuessler WW, Vancaillie TG, Reich H, Griffith DP (1991) Transperitoneal endosurgical lymphadenectomy in patients with localized prostate cancer. J Urol 145:988
7. Griffith DP, Schuessler WW, Nickell KG, Meaney JT (1992) Laparoscopic pelvic lymphadenectomy for prostatic adenocarcinoma. Urol Clin North Am 19:407–415
8. Kerbl K, Clayman RV, Petros JA, Chandhoke PS, Gill IS (1993) Staging pelvic lymphadenectomy for prostate cancer: a comparison of laparoscopic and open techniques. J Urol 150:396–399
9. Parra RO, Andrus C, Boullier J (1992) Staging laparoscopic pelvic lymph node dissection: comparison of results with open pelvic lymphadenectomy. J Urol 147:875–878
10. Moore RG, Partin AW, Kavoussi LR (1996) Role of laparoscopy in the diagnosis and treatment of prostate cancer. Sem Surg Oncol 12:139–144
11. Arcangeli CG, Ornstein DK, Keetch DW, Andriole GL (1997) Prostate specific antigen as a screening test for prostate cancer. The United States experience. Urol Clin North Am 24:299
12. Catalona WJ, Smith DS, Ornstein DK (1997) Prostate cancer detection in men with serum PSA concentrations of 2.6 to 4.0 ng/ml. and benign prostate examination. Enhancement of specificity with free PSA measurements. JAMA 227:11452
13. Keetch DW, Catalona WJ, Smith DS (1994) Serial prostatic biopsies in men with persistently elevated serum prostate specific antigen values. J Urol 151:1571
14. Petros JA, Catalona WJ (1992) Lower incidence of unsuspected lymph node metastases in 521 consecutive patients with clinically localized prostate cancer. J Urol 147:1574–1575
15. Danella JF, Dekernion JB, Smith RB, Steckel J (1993) The contemporary incidence of lymph node metastases in prostate cancer: implications for laparoscopic lymph node dissection. J Urol 149:1488–1491
16. Partin AW, Yoo J, Carter HB, Pearson JD, Chan DW, Epstein JI, Walsh PC (1993) The use of prostate specific antigen, clinical stage, and Gleason score to predict pathological stage in men with localized prostate cancer. J Urol 150:110–114
17. Partin AW, Kattan MW, Subong EN, Walsh PC, Wojno KJ, Osterling JE, Scardino PT, Person JD (1997) Combination of prostate-specific antigen, clinical stage, and Gleason score to predict pathological stage of localized prostate cancer. A multi-institutional update. JAMA 277:1445
18. Sands ME, Zagars GK, Pollack A, von Eschenback AC (1994) Serum prostate specific antigen, clinical stage, pathologic grade, and the incidence of nodal metastases in prostate cancer. Urology 44:215–220
19. Roach M, Marquez C, Yuo H-S (1993) Predicting the risk of lymph node involvement using pretreatment prostate specific antigen and Gleason score in men with clinically localized prostate cancer. Int J Radiation Oncol Biol Phys 28:33–37

20. Kava BR, Dalbagni G, Conlon KC, Russo P (1998) Results of laparoscopic pelvic lymphadenectomy in patients at high risk for nodal metastases from prostate cancer. Ann Surg Oncol 5:173–180

21. Stone NA, Stock RG, Unger P (1995) Indications for seminal vesicle biopsy and laparoscopic pelvic lymph node dissection in men with localized carcinoma of the prostate. J Urol 154:1392

22. Stone NN, Stock RG, Parikh D, Yeghiayan P, Unger P (1998) Perineural invasion and seminal vesicle involvement predict pelvic lymph node metastasis in men with localized carcinoma of the prostate. J Urol 160:1722–1726

23. Winfield HN, Donovan JF, See WA, Loening SA, Williams RD (1992) Laparoscopic pelvic lymph node dissection for genitourinary malignancies: indications techniques, and results. J Endourol 6:103

24. Donat SM, Herr HW, Bajorin DR, Fair WR, Sogani PC, Russo P, Sheinfeld J, Scher HI (1996) Methotrexate, vinblastine, doxorubicin and cisplatin chemotherapy and cystectomy for unresectable bladder cancer. J Urol 156:368–371

25. Kava BR, Russo P, Conlon KC (1996) Laparoscopic diagnosis of malignant retroperitoneal fibrosis. J Endourol 10:535–538

26. Gerber GS, Rukstalis DB (1996) Laparoscopic approach to retroperitoneal lymph node dissection. Sem Surg Oncol 12:121–125

27. Janetschek G, Hobisch A, Holtl L, Bartsch G (1996) Retroperitoneal lymphadenectomy for clinical stage 1 nonseminomatous testicular tumor: Laparoscopic versus open surgery and the impact of the learning curve. J Urol 156:89–93

28. Hulbert JC, Fraley EE (1992) Laparoscopic retroperitoneal lymphadenectomy. New approach to staging clinical stage 1 germ cell tumors of the testis. J Endourol 6:123

29. Moore R, Rosenberg MT, O'Donnell MA, Kavoussi LR (1993) Laparoscopic retroperitoneal lymph node sampling (LRPNS). J Endourol 7:S170

30. Peters CA, Kavoussi LR, Retik AB (1993) Laparoscopic management of the intra abdominal testis. J Endourol 7:S170

31. Cortes D, Thorup JM, Lenz K, Beck BL, Nielsen OH (1995) Laparoscopy in 100 consecutive patients with 128 impalpable testes. Br J Urol 75:281–287

32. Russo P, Grimaldi G, Conlon KC (1998) Laparoscopic resection of intra-abdominal testicular tumor. Urology 51:122–124

33. Mukai M, Takamatsu H, Noguchi H, Tahara H (1998) Intra-abdominal testis with mature teratoma. Pediatr Surg Int 13:204–205

34. Gill IS, Kerbl K, Clayman RV (1993) Laparoscopic surgery in urology: Current applications. AJR160:1167–1170

35. Kerbl K, Clayman RV, McDougall EM, Kavoussi LR (1994) Laparoscopic nephrectomy: the Washington University experience. Br J Urol 73:231–236

36. McDougall EM, Clayman RV, Elashry O (1995) Laparoscopic nephroureterectomy for upper tract transitional cell carcinoma: The Washington University experience. J Urol 154:975–980

37. Kavoussi LR, Kerbl K, Capelouto CC, McDougall EM, Clayman RV (1993) Laparoscopic nephrectomy for renal neoplasms. Urology 42:603–608

38. Gill IS, Kavoussi LR, Clayman RV et al. (1995) Complications of laparoscopic nephrectomy in 185 patients: A multi-institutional review. J Urol 154:479–483

39. Motzer RJ, Russo P, Nanus DM, Berg WJ (1997) Renal cell carcinoma. Curr Probl in Cancer 121:185–232

40. Licht MR, Novick AC, Goormastic M (1994) Nephron sparing surgery in incidental versus suspected renal cell carcinoma. J Urol 152:39–42

41. Moll V, Becht E, Ziegler M (1993) Kidney preserving surgery in renal cell tumors: Indications, techniques, and results in 152 patients. J Urol 150:319–323
42. Winfield HN, Donovan JF, Lund GO, Kreder KJ, Stanley KE, Brown BP, Loening SA, Clayman RV (1995) Laparoscopic partial nephrectomy: Initial experience and comparison to the open surgical approach. J Urol 153:1409–1414
43. Kerbl K, Clayman RV (1994) Advances in laparoscopic renal and ureteral surgery. Eur Urol 25:1–6
44. Hayakawa K, Nishiyama T, Ohashi M, Ishikawa H, Hata M (1997) A trial of laparoscopic assisted radical nephrectomy. Jap J Urol 88:801–806
45. Nishiyama T, Terunuma M (1995) Laparoscopy-assisted radical nephrectomy in combination with minilaparotomy: report of initial 7 cases. Int J Urol 2:124–127
46. Santiago L, Yamaguchi R, Kaswick J, Bellman GC (1998) Laparoscopic management of indeterminant renal cysts. Urology 52:379–383

Is There Any Role for the Laparoscopic Staging of Urologic Malignancies?

P. Fornara · C. Doehn · D. Jocham

▌ Introduction

Preoperative or intraoperative staging is often necessary in urologic malignancies to plan further treatment modalities. Various imaging techniques are used, but results are often unsatisfactory. New minimally invasive approaches like laparoscopy may change staging and treatment strategies in patients with urologic malignancies.

Cortesi introduced laparoscopic urology in 1976 for the evaluation of the non-palpable testis [1]. Laparoscopy for cryptorchidism, however, remained a diagnostic procedure and the only laparoscopic procedure within urology for a long time. In 1989, Schuessler and colleagues performed the first laparoscopic pelvic lymphadenectomy on a patient with prostate cancer [2]. Since then, laparoscopy has been used for many urologic diseases but only a few indications have survived to be generally accepted (Tables 1–3).

Laparoscopy is believed to be associated with obvious clinical benefits for the patient in terms of less morbidity, less pain and analgesic consumption, shorter hospital stay, and briefer convalescence [3–6]. In certain conditions such as cryptorchidism or bilateral varicoceles, technical advantages of laparoscopy exist compared with other surgical techniques and may support the indication for this minimally invasive technique. In a recent survey of urologists in the USA, the most common laparoscopic procedure performed is pelvic lymphadenectomy in patients with prostate cancer.

Table 1. Indications for laparoscopy (American Urological Association, AUA 1996)

Clear indications	Possible indications	Doubtful indications
Cryptorchidism	Suspension	Varicocele resection
Lymphocele resection	Retroperitoneal LAD	Prostatectomy
Nephrectomy for benign disease	Pyeloplasty	Cystectomy
Pelvic lymphadenectomy (LAD)	Adrenalectomy	Kidney donation
	Nephrectomy for malignancy	
	Heminephrectomy	

Table 2. Indications for laparoscopy (German Urological Association, DGU 1994)

Clear indications
Nephrectomy for benign disease
Nephroureterectomy for benign disease
Cryptorchidism
Adrenalectomy
Lymphocele resection
Renal cyst resection
Varicocele resection (relapse or bilateral)

Table 3. Indications for laparoscopy in patients with urologic malignancy (German Urological Association, DGU 1995)

Malignancy	Indication for laparoscopy?
Prostate cancer	Only in few patients
TCC[a]	No
Renal cancer	No
Testicular cancer	Only experimental
Penile cancer	No

[a]Transitional cell carcinoma of the bladder and upper urinary tract.

In this chapter the most common urologic malignancies [prostate cancer, transitional cell carcinoma (TCC) of the bladder and upper urinary tract, renal cancer, testicular cancer, and penile cancer] are described according to their characteristics, preoperative staging, treatment modalities, and the potential role of laparoscopy in staging.

▌Prostate Cancer

Prostate cancer is the second most common cancer in men, accounting for 334,500 new cases in the USA in 1997. The most important risk factors are age, positive family history, and race. More than 50% of these patients are older than 65. It is known that 15%–30% of men older than 50 years and 80% of patients older than 80 have histopathological signs of prostate cancer. However, only 10% of these patients will ever have clinical evidence of prostate cancer. The preoperative staging and treatment modalities are given in Tables 4 and 5.

Because either radical prostatectomy or radiotherapy can cure organ-confined cancer it is essential to exclude metastases. Usually, the first occurrence of tumor spread is detected in the pelvic lymph nodes. Therefore, a histopathological examination of these lymph nodes is of prognostic and therapeutic relevance.

Table 4. Preoperative staging of prostate cancer

Digital rectal examination (DRE)
Tumor marker (PSA[a])
Transrectal ultrasound (TRUS)
Intravenous urogram (IVU)
Urethrocystogram (UCG)
Cystoscopy
Chest X-ray
Bone scan[b]
Computed tomography
Magnetic resonance imaging (endorectal surface coil)

[a]Prostate specific antigen.
[b]Only when PSA greater than 10 ng/ml.

Table 5. Therapy of prostate cancer

Therapy	Characteristics and limitations
Radical prostatectomy (retropubic or perineal) after pelvic lymphadenectomy	Only for localized disease, only when life expectancy is of 10 years or more, impotence(50%–100%) and incontinence (5%–40%)
Radiotherapy (external beam or implant radiation therapy)	Curative intention but less successful (10-year survival rate) than radical prostatectomy for localized disease
Antiandrogen therapy (surgical or medical castration	In advanced stages. May delay time to progression but not survival rates
Surveillance patient compliance necessary	Only in T1G1 disease, close follow-up and
Chemotherapy (e.g., estramustin phosphate, mitomycin	Only palliative, second-line therapy with low response rates
Symptomatic therapy (e.g., analgesics, radiotherapy of bone metastases	Only palliative to improve symptoms

Technique of Laparoscopic Pelvic Lymphadenectomy

The patient is placed in a supine position under general anesthesia in a 30° head-down position. After induction of anesthesia, a nasogastric tube and a bladder catheter are placed to decompress the stomach and bladder.

One should start on the side where positive nodes are expected, otherwise on the right side. Four or five ports are necessary for laparoscopic lymph node dissection. After creation of the pneumoperitoneum an incision of the peritoneum from the internal inguinal ring to the bifurcation of the common iliac artery lateral to the medial umbilical ligament (=obliterated umbilical arteries) is performed. Landmarks are the umbilical ligament (medial), the pubic bone (anterior), and the external iliac vessels (lateral).

The spermatic cord and vas deferens are ligated to expose the iliac-obturator space. Preparation of the lymph nodes is performed from caudal to cranial with careful sparing of the obturator nerve. The lymph nodes can be removed through a port, and the procedure is repeated on the contralateral side. The peritoneum is usually not closed.

▌ Testicular Cancer

Testicular cancer accounts for 1%–2% of all cancers in men. In 1997, 7,200 new cases occurred in the USA and 2,600 new cases were reported in Germany. More than 90% of patients can be cured. The most frequent tumors are germ cell tumors like seminomas (40%) and nonseminomas (35%). Approximately 70% of all patients are between 20 and 40, and the mean age is 26 years for patients with nonseminoma and 36 years for patients with seminoma. The incidence of testicular cancer is high in the Western world and low in Asia and Africa. The most important risk factor is the undescended testicle, with a five- to tenfold elevated risk

Table 6. Preoperative staging of testicular cancer

Ultrasound
Tumor marker (AFP, HCG, LDH, HPLAP)
Chest X-ray
Computed tomography
Bone scan

AFP, Alpha-fetoprotein; HCG, human chorionic gonadotropin; LDH, lactate dehydrogenase; HPLAP, human placental alkaline phosphatase.

Table 7. Therapy of testicular cancer

Stage	Seminoma	Nonseminoma
First step	Inguinal orchiectomy and contralateral biopsy	Inguinal orchiectomy and contralateral biopsy
Second step		
Stage I	Radiotherapy (26 Gy) or chemotherapy (experimental)	Retroperitoneal lymphadenectomy or surveillance
Stage IIa/b	Radiotherapy (30--36 Gy) or chemotherapy (experimental) nodes	Retroperitoneal lymphadenectomy, chemotherapy in case of positive
Stage IIc/III	Chemotherapy	Chemotherapy

or 2% chance of developing testicular cancer by the age of 65. Other risk factors are Klinefelter syndrome or a history of mumps orchitis. The preoperative staging and treatment modalities are given in Tables 6 and 7.

It is widely accepted that patients with clinical stage I nonseminoma are candidates for retroperitoneal lymphadenectomy, because this tumor spreads into these nodes and imaging studies give 30% false negative results in these patients. Vice versa, 70% of these patients have no lymph node metastases when undergoing retroperitoneal lymphadenectomy. Therefore, an alternative approach is surveillance (e.g., in patients with negative tumor markers) with close follow-up studies.

Technique of Laparoscopic Retroperitoneal Lymphadenectomy

The Veress needle is placed supraumbilically, and two 12-mm trocars are placed along the midclavicular line just below the costal margin and approximately 5 cm below the umbilicus. Two 5-mm trocars are placed along the ipsilateral anterior auxiliary line. One is placed just above the ileal crest parallel to the umbilicus and the other just below the costal margin. With the endoscissors, an incision into the ipsilateral line of Toldt is made. The bowel is retracted medially, and the retroperitoneum is inspected. If gross disease is noted, this should be biopsied, and when positive for a tumor in the frozen section, the procedure should be continued in an open fashion. In case of the absence of bulky disease, laparoscopy should be continued with identification of the ipsilateral spermatic cord. The cord is mobilized distally to the internal inguinal ring and proximally to the aortic bifurcation. The spermatic vein is ligated at the level of the inguinal ring and renal vein. Then the ureter is mobilized followed by the removal of Gerota's fascia from the renal capsule. The nodal tissue is gently teased from around the large vessels from cranial to caudal. Careful dissection along the aorta will expose the sympathetic nerve fibers, which can be easily seen with laparoscopic magnification. The lymph node package is removed via a 12-mm trocar using an entrapment sac.

Role of Laparoscopy for Staging of Transitional Cell Carcinoma of the Bladder and Upper Urinary Tract

Bladder cancer represents 3%–4% of all tumors, with 52,900 new cases in the USA and 10,400 in Germany in 1996. The age at diagnosis is between 65 and 75 years in most cases, with a male-to-female ratio of 3:1. The highest rates are found in the Western world, whereas the lowest rates are found in developing countries in Asia. The strongest risk factors are smoking, analgesic abuse, and industry-related carcinogens (e.g., aromatic amines). Approximately 90% of all malignant bladder tumors are TCC arising from the urothelium. Superficial stages (Ta/T1/CIS) are present in 70%–90% of patients at initial presentation with relapse rates between 30% and 90% within 3 years. However, progression to higher and muscle-invasive stages (T2/T3/T4) may occur in 4%–32% depending on

Table 8. Preoperative staging of transitional cell carcinoma of the bladder and upper urinary tract

Ultrasound
Intravenous urogram (IVU)
Chest X-ray
Computed tomography[a]
Bone scan

[a]In case of muscle-invasive tumor (histology with T2 stage or more).

Table 9. Therapy of bladder cancer

Stage	Therapy
CIS/Ta/T1 (superficial tumor)	TUR and prophylaxis (instillation of BCG, mitomycin, or doxorubicin, photodynamic therapy)
T2/T3 (muscle-invasive tumor)	Radical cystectomy with LAD and urinary diversion (e.g., neobladder, pouch, ileal conduit), palliative TUR-B
T4 (advanced tumor)	Palliative cystectomy, chemotherapy and/or radiotherapy, palliative TUR-B, or symptomatic therapy

stage, therapy, and follow-up studies. Metastasis from superficial bladder cancer may develop in less than 1% from Ta tumors but 22% from T1G3 tumors. In up to 10% of patients with TCC the upper urinary tract is involved. In these patients, endoscopic resection, partial resection of the ureter, or radical nephroureterectomy with lymphadenectomy is applied according to tumor stage. Preoperative staging and therapy modalities are given in Tables 8 and 9.

Renal Cancer

Renal cancer represents 2%–3% of all cancers, accounting for 30,600 new cases in the USA in 1996. In 75% of all patients the age at diagnosis is between 60 and 75 years, with a male-to-female ratio of 2:1. The highest rates are found in Scandinavia, whereas the lowest rates are found in Japan. The strongest risk factors are smoking, analgesic abuse, and obesity. Acquired renal cystic disease is a risk factor only in end-stage renal disease. Hereditary forms of renal cell carcinoma exist with an autosomal dominant transmission.

Most cases are adenocarcinomas (80%–90%) arising from proximal tubular cells. Metastases develop by lymphatic spread or hematogenous spread into the lung, liver, bone, or brain. Since the introduction of ultrasound, renal cancer is often detected at earlier stages; however, 20%–30% of all patients still have metas-

Table 10. Preoperative staging of renal cancer

Ultrasound
Intravenous urogram (IVU)
Chest X-ray
Computed tomography
Angiography
Bone scan

Table 11. Therapy of renal cancer

Stage	Therapy
T1/T2	Partial nephrectomy or radical nephrectomy with LAD and adrenalectomy (for upper pole tumors)
T3	Radical nephrectomy with LAD and adrenalectomy
T4 (advanced tumor)	Palliative nephrectomy, immunotherapy (in combination with chemotherapy), and/or symptomatic therapy

tases at initial presentation.

Node involvement, T stage, and presence of metastases are the most important prognostic factors. Relapse occurs within 3 years after diagnosis in most cases. Five-year survival in patients is 90% with T1 tumors and decreases with higher T stages (75% for T2, 55% for T3, and 5% for T4). Patients with metastases have a life expectancy of 6–18 months.

Most of the regional lymph nodes of the kidney are in the hilum around the renal artery and vein as well as vena cava and aorta. Because tumor removal is the only therapy with a curative intention, staging lymphadenectomy before tumor removal is not indicated in patients with renal cancer. Apart from staging aspects, however, laparoscopic nephrectomy for renal cell carcinoma is frequently performed in the USA and Japan, whereas in Germany this procedure is generally not recommended. Preoperative staging and treatment modalities are given in Tables 10 and 11.

Penile Cancer

Penile cancer accounts for 0.4%–0.6% of all tumors in men in the Western world, with 950 new cases in the USA in 1996. The typical age is between 60 and 80 years. The disease has been reported in all races but is more common in Asia, Africa, and South America (up to 10% of all tumors). Social and cultural habits seem to be more important than racial factors in penile cancer. Phimosis (75% of patients with penile cancer have a history of phimosis), poor hygiene, and photochemotherapy (PUVA) for psoriasis are associated with this tumor. Penile cancer can be associated with HPV infection; predominantly HPV type 16 has been found in such patients. Circumcision in newborns gives nearly 100% protection against the disease.

Most cases are squamous cell tumors (95%) arising from the glans or inner surface of the foreskin. Metastases develop by lymphatic spread [between Scarpa's fascia and fascia lata (superficial nodes), between fascia lata and femoral vein (deep inguinal nodes), and external iliac nodes in the pelvis]. Fifty percent of patients present enlarged nodes [physical examination or computed tomography (CT) scan], but only 30% will have metastases. Another 10%–15% of patients with initial N0 will develop lymph node metastases during follow-up. Although nodal metastases are relatively common, distant dissemination is very rare.

Most relapses occur within 3 years after diagnosis. Node involvement is the most important prognostic factor. Five-year survival is 85%–100% in patients with negative nodes, 17%–75% in patients with positive nodes, and only 15% in patients not treated with lymphadenectomy. Preoperative staging and treatment modalities are given in Tables 12 and 13.

Table 12. Preoperative staging of penile cancer

Ultrasound (US)
Tumoral marker (SCC[a])
Chest X-ray
Computed tomography (facultative)
Bone scan (facultative)
sentinel node (facultative)

[a]Squamous cell carcinoma antigen

Table 13. Therapy of penile cancer

Stage	Therapy
First step	
CIS/T1	Circumcision, laser and/or radiotherapy, and/or partial penectomy
T2	Partial penectomy
T3	Total penectomy
T4	Emasculation
Second step	
Low risk	Inguinal LAD or surveillance
High risk	Inguinal (and pelvic) LAD
Third step	
Negative nodes	Surveillance
Positive nodes	Chemotherapy

Discussion

Laparoscopic urology is an expanding field, and new materials, instruments, and procedures continue to evolve. Despite the great advances witnessed over the past years, the ultimate role for laparoscopy in urology is still being defined. Laparoscopic pelvic lymphadenectomy has gained acceptance for the staging of pelvic malignancies, primarily for prostate cancer. Ablative procedures removing organs with malignant tumors have received less enthusiasm for a number of reasons. There are fears of tumor spillage and inadequate tumor margins [7–9]. However, port site metastasis has been most often reported in patients with colorectal cancer, ovarian cancer, and cancer of the gallbladder [7]. Port site metastasis after laparoscopic lymphadenectomy for prostatic or bladder cancer is less common, with only a few cases reported in the literature [8, 9]. Higher technical demands and longer operative times compared with open surgical techniques are present in certain laparoscopic operations.

Laparoscopic procedures for removal or staging of almost all urologic tumors have been performed and reported as single case reports or small series. However, it is of importance that the American Association of Urologists (Table 1) has recommended laparoscopic lymphadenectomy only in patients with prostate cancer. The German Urological Association has recommended laparoscopy only for laparoscopic pelvic lymphadenectomy in patients with prostate cancer who have an increased risk of lymph node involvement but not for any other patients with urologic malignancies (Table 3).

Current imaging studies such as CT, magnetic resonance imaging (MRI), ultrasound, and pelvic lymphangiography assess the pathological stage of pelvic lymph nodes poorly. Accurate staging of pelvic or retroperitoneal lymph nodes is essential in patients with cancer of the prostate, bladder, upper urinary tract, testicle, and penis. Because lymphadenectomy can be performed in an open manner one must question whether laparoscopy is superior to open surgery.

Role of Laparoscopy for Staging of Prostate Cancer

The importance of determining the presence of lymph node involvement from prostate cancer, or any other urologic malignancy, is that the finding will most likely determine the extent of treatment and the feasibility of curative therapy. In most urologic centers, the detection of positive nodes from prostate cancer would negate the possibility for radical prostatectomy with curative intention. At this point, the patient would be offered the options of surgical or medical castration or observation until the malignancy became symptomatic. Absence of positive lymph nodes would allow urologists to offer a retropubic or perineal prostatectomy or external or interstitial radiotherapy, with curative intention. Therefore, the indication for laparoscopic lymphadenectomy is given before planned radiotherapy, perineal prostatectomy, or radical retropubic prostatectomy when lymph node involvement is suspected [e.g., prostate-specific antiven (PSA) greater than 20 ng/ml, Gleason score greater than 7, and/or suspicious nodes in CT scan].

It is well documented that pelvic lymph node metastasis, even when minimal, indicate a poor prognosis regardless of the treatment modality used. Lymph node involvement is evident in 5%–30% of patients with localized prostate cancer. Can positive nodes be predicted by better parameters than imaging studies? When PSA is between 20 and 50 ng/ml the chance of positive nodes is 65% [10]. In another study, a PSA greater than 20 ng/ml was the single best prognostic parameter to predict positive lymph nodes with a 40% chance [11]. Other parameters were high clinical stage, large size of the prostate, and a Gleason score of more than 7 obtained from prostate biopsy before radical surgery [11]. On the other hand, Bluestein and Narayan found 97% and 99%, respectively, of patients with a PSA less than 10 ng/ml to have negative pelvic lymph nodes [12, 13]. Generally, prostate cancer is detected earlier now because of improved diagnostic tools. Pelvic lymphadenectomy remains, however, the only accurate method capable of determining the status of the pelvic lymph nodes in prostate cancer patients. Presently, pelvic lymph node dissection can be performed by either an open or a laparoscopic approach as detailed in Table 14 [14–31]. The combination of laparoscopic pelvic lymph node dissection with radical perineal prostatecto-

Table 14. Laparoscopic staging of prostate cancer: review of the literature[a]

Author and year	Patients (n)	Mean OP time (min)	Lymph nodes (n)	Morbidity rate (%)
Schuessler 1991 [2]	12	510	14.7	8.3
Kavoussi 1993 [14]	372	Not given	Not given	15
Schuessler 1993 [15]	147	150	45.3	31
Burney 1993 [16]	49	160	Not given	35.1
Kerbl 1993 [17]	30	199	Not given	13
Rukstalis 1994 [18]	94	156	6.9	13.5
Guazzoni 1994 [19]	30	136	17.5	23
Levy 1994 [20]	37	244[b]	Not given	Not given
Parra 1994 [21]	76	244[b]	Not given	Not given
Schoborg 1994 [22]	50	Not given	Not given	8
Maffezzini 1995 [23]	158	Not given	11	16
Stone 1995 [24]	130	226[b]	Not given	67.1[b]
Klän 1995 [25]	70	Not given	13.6	24.3
Brant 1996 [26]	60	120	10	6.7
Effert 1996 [27]	120	120	11	10
Parra 1996 [28]	40	55	Not given	Not given
Cadeddu 1997 [29]	52	Not given	9.8	7.7
Fahlenkamp 1997 [30]	200	110	11	11.5
Hoenig 1997 [31]	120	Not given	Not given	Not given

[a]Only series with more than 30 patients.
[b]Combined with radical surgery.

my overcomes the distinct disadvantage of lack of access to the pelvic lymph nodes classically connected with the perineal approach while at the same time avoiding an abdominal incision. Open lymph node dissection is associated with morbidity (up to 35%) including vascular and neurological injuries, lymphocele formation, and deep vein thrombosis as well as postoperative medical complications [32, 33]. Laparoscopic lymph node dissection is also not devoid of risks (Table 14). A combined laparoscopic and sentinel approach to detect lymphatic spread must be evaluated in the future.

Another plus for the two-step procedure (first step: laparoscopic pelvic lymphadenectomy; second step: perineal or retropubic lymphadenectomy) is that frozen sections have false negative rates up to 41.7% and final histology can be awaited before perineal prostatectomy is performed [34, 35].

Currently, one must state that retropubic and perineal prostatectomy are comparable in terms of tumor control. When retropubic prostatectomy is performed, pelvic lymphadenectomy is integrated into the operation, whereas in patients with a high risk of having positive lymph nodes, laparoscopy before radical surgery might be of benefit. Patients undergoing perineal prostatectomy should undergo laparoscopic pelvic lymphadenectomy with prostatectomy during the same session or as a second-step procedure.

Role of Laparoscopy for Staging of Testicular Cancer

For patients with low-stage nonseminomatous testicular tumors, open retroperitoneal node dissection is often required for accurate staging as well as for therapeutic purposes. However, the morbidity associated with open surgery has stimulated research into more limited surgical dissection or surveillance protocols with no surgery. This disease was initially treated with aggressive bilateral retroperitoneal lymph node dissections. Dissection was done bilaterally above the renal hilum. The morbidity of this procedure was high and included complete ejaculatory impotence. Donohue and colleagues developed less morbid surgery for this disease including only the dissection of the area of the ipsilateral lymph node area. To minimize the damage to the preaortic autonomic nerves supplying the ejaculatory system, the dissection of retroperitoneal lymph nodes below the inferior mesenteric artery is limited to the ipsilateral side. Almost all metastases of left-sided testicular tumors occur in the left para-aortic and preaortic region, whereas right-sided tumors predominantly spread to the interaortocaval, precaval, and paracaval region and lateral the common iliac artery.

One of the more advanced laparoscopic procedures performed in urology is the retroperitoneal lymph node dissection for stage I nonseminomatous testicular cancer. Such a procedure is feasible in skilled and experienced hands, but its ultimate role in the staging and treatment of testis tumors must be defined. Conversely, a well-performed open retroperitoneal lymph node dissection is effective as a staging tool and is known to be curative in almost all patients with pathological stage I and more than 50% of stage II cases.

The largest series of laparoscopic RPLND reports a 30% complication rate, with bleeding being the most common event (Table 15). The major difficulty entails controlling and dissecting the lumbar vessels. Because dissection posterior

Table 15. Laparoscopic staging of testicular cancer: review of the literature

Author and year	Patients (n)	Stage	Mean OP time (min)	Lymph-nodes (n)	Morbidity-rate (%, event)
Rukstalis 1992 [36]	1	1	510	28	Blood transfusion
Gerber 1994 [37]	20	1	360	14.5	30% (Bleeding, conversions)
Janetschek 1996 [38]	29	I or II	452	Not given	17% (Conversion, lymphocele, lymph edema, pressure sores)
Rassweiler 1996 [39]	26	I or II	298	12	21% (Ureteral stenosis, pulmonary embolism, retrograde ejaculation)

to the large vessels is not yet possible, this approach can not claim the same therapeutic benefit as the classical open approach. Follow-up is short, and the completeness of the dissection is unknown because the patients were not operated in an open fashion except for surgical complications. Despite the prolonged operative time of 4–6 h, the major advantages of laparoscopic RPLND are realized in the postoperative period. This technique has been performed only in a small number of patients, and its role still has to be defined.

Role of Laparoscopy for Staging of Transitional Cell Carcinoma of the Bladder and Upper Urinary Tract

With the realization that pelvic lymphadenectomy in combination with radical cystectomy did not significantly increase the mortality or morbidity compared with cystectomy alone but also improved the clinical staging and survival of patients with micrometastases in a single or a few nodes, most urologic surgeons now advocate this radical approach. In most patients there is no need for sole lymphadenectomy either open or laparoscopically. However, laparoscopic lymphadenectomy might be considered in patients who refuse cystectomy and desire definitive radiotherapy, patients being considered for partial cystectomy, or patients with aggressive bladder cancer, where, in the presence of positive nodes, cystectomy would not be curative (Table 16). Patients with TCC of the upper urinary tract do not benefit from laparoscopic staging; however, laparoscopic nephroureterectomy for malignancy is an established procedure in the USA and other countries.

Table 16. Laparoscopic staging of bladder cancer: review of the literature

Author and year (n)	Patients (min)	Mean OP time (n)	Lymph nodes (%, event)	Morbidity
Bowsher 1992 [40]	2	110	Not given	None
Ovesen 1993 [41]	54	360	Not given	???
Villers 1993 [42]	8	84	Not given	12.5% (Sepsis)
Burney 1993 [16]	3	160	Not given	33% (Bladder injury)
Prasad 1994 [43]	1	140	5	None
Lang 1994 [44]	2	Not given	9.3	None
Puppo 1994 [45]	13	145	12.4	53.8 (Pain, subcutaneous emphysema)
Poulsen 1995 [46]	19	120	5	16% (Port hernia, bleeding, hematoma, conversion)

Conclusions

Laparoscopic lymphadenectomy in patients with urologic malignancies is technically feasible and safe. However, the technique is only indicated in a few patients with clinically organ-confined prostate cancer or low-stage nonseminomatous testicular cancer.

In patients with prostate cancer scheduled for a retropubic prostatectomy, only those with a high susceptibility of pelvic lymph node involvement are candidates for laparoscopy. In patients scheduled for perineal prostatectomy or radiotherapy, there is an obvious technical advantage in performing a laparoscopic pelvic lymphadenectomy as a first step. Operative times and results are comparable to those for an open pelvic lymphadenectomy.

Patients with low-stage nonseminomatous testicular cancer undergoing retroperitoneal lymphadenectomy may profit from the laparoscopic approach in terms of a briefer postoperative course. However, laparoscopic retroperitoneal lymphadenectomy requires much longer operative times, and the therapeutic benefit for these patients is still being debated. Therefore, this procedure is still experimental.

Patients with TCC of the bladder and upper urinary tract, renal cancer, or penile cancer are generally not candidates for staging laparoscopy because the diagnostic benefit is low, as illustrated in Table 17.

Table 17. Value of laparoscopic staging for urologic malignancies

Malignancy	Experimental value	Clinical value
Prostate cancer	+	±
TCC[a]	–	–
Renal cancer	–	–
Testicular cancer	±	–
Penile cancer	–	–

[a]Transitional cell carcinoma of the bladder and upper urinary tract.

▌ References

1. Cortesi N, Ferrari P, Zambarda E, Mananti E, Baldini E, Pignate Morano F (1976) Diagnosis of bilateral abdominal cryptorchidism by laparoscopy. Endoscopy 8:33–34
2. Schuessler WW, Vancaillie TG, Reich H, Griffith DP (1991) Transperitoneal endosurgical lymphadenectomy in patients with localized prostate cancer. J Urol 145:988–991
3. Fornara P, Doehn C, Fricke L, Durek C, Thyssen G, Jocham D (1997) Laparoscopic bilateral nephrectomy: results in 11 renal transplant patients. J Urol 157:445–449
4. Doehn C, Fornara P, Jocham D (1998) Comparison of laparoscopic and open nephrectomy for benign renal conditions. Eur Urol 33 [Suppl 1]:38
5. Doehn C, Fornara P, Jocham D (1998) Comparison of laparoscopic and open nephroureterectomy for benign disease. J Urol 159:732–734
6. Fornara P, Doehn C, Jocham D (1997) Systemic response after laparoscopic and open nephrectomy: results from prospective controlled animal and clinical studies. J Urol 157:139
7. Nduka CC, Monson JRT, Menzies-Gow N, Darzi A (1994) Abdominal wall metastases following laparoscopy. Br J Surg 81:648–652
8. Bangma CH, Kirkels WJ, Chadha S, Schröder FH (1995) Cutaneous metastasis following laparoscopic pelvic lymphadenectomy for prostatic carcinoma. J Urol 153:1635–1636
9. Elbahnasy AM, Hoenig DM, Shalav A, McDougall EM, Clayman RV (1998) Laparoscopic staging of bladder tumor: concerns about port site metastases. J Endourol 12:55–59
10. Hudson MA, Bahnson RR, Catalona WJ (1989) Clinical use of prostate specific antigen in patients with prostate cancer. J Urol 142:1011–1017
11. Parra RO, Isorna S, Garcia Perez M, Cummings JM, Boullier JA (1996) Radical perineal prostatectomy without lymphadenectomy: selection criteria and early results. J Urol 155:612–615
12. Bluestein DL, Bostwick DG, Bergstralh EJ, Oesterling JE (1994) Eliminating the need for bilateral pelvic lymphadenectomy in select patients with prostate cancer. J Urol 151:1315–1320
13. Narayan P, Fournier G, Gajendran V, Leidich R, Lo R, Wolf JS Jr, Jakob G, Nicolaisen G, Palmer K, Freiha F (1994) Utility of preoperative serum prostate-specific antigen concentration and biopsy Gleason score in predicting risk of pelvic lymph node metastases in prostate cancer. Urology 44:519–524
14. Kavoussi LR, Sosa E, Chandhoke P, Chodak G, Clayman RV, Hadley R, Loughlin KR, Ruckle HC, Rukstalis D, Schuessler W, Segura J, Vancaillie T, Winfield HN (1993) Complications of laparoscopic pelvic lymph node dissection. J Urol 149:322–325

15. Schuessler WW, Pharand D, Vancaillie TG (1993) Laparoscopic standard pelvic node dissection for carcinoma of the prostate: is it accurate? J Urol 150:898–901
16. Burney TL, Campbell Jr EC, Naslund MJ, Jacobs SC (1993) Complications of staging laparoscopic pelvic lymphadenectomy. Surg Laparosc Endosc 3:184–190
17. Kerbl K, Clayman RV, Petros JA, Chandhoke PS, Gill IS (1993) Staging pelvic lymphadenectomy for prostate cancer: comparison of laparoscopic and open techniques. J Urol 150:396–399
18. Rukstalis DB, Gerber GS, Vogelzang NJ, Haraf DJ, Straus II FH, Chodak GW (1994) Laparoscopic pelvic lymph node dissection: a review of 103 consecutive cases. J Urol 151:670–674
19. Guazzoni G, Montrosi F, Bergamaschi F, Bellinzoni P, Centemero A, Consonni P, Rigatti P (1994) Open surgical revision of laparoscopic pelvic lymphadenectomy for staging of prostate cancer: the impact of laparoscopic learning curve. J Urol 151:930–933
20. Levy DA, Resnick MI (1994) Laparoscopic pelvic lymphadenectomy and radical perineal prostatectomy: a viable alternative to radical retropubic prostatectomy. J Urol 151:905–908
21. Parra RO, Boullier JA, Rauscher JA, Cummings JM (1994) The value of laparoscopic lymphadenectomy in conjunction with radical perineal or retropubic prostatectomy. J Urol 151:1599–1602
22. Schoborg TW (1994) Laparoscopic staging of prostatic carcinoma. Semin Surg Oncol 10:422–430
23. Maffezzini M, Carmignani G, Perachino M, Puppo P, Montorsi F, Guazzoni G, Gallucci M, Di Silverio F, Morelli M, Muto G (1995) Benefits and complications of laparoscopic pelvic lymphadenectomy for detection of stage D1 prostate cancer: a multicenter experience. Eur Urol 27:135–137
24. Stone NN, Ramin SA, Wesson MF, Stock R, Unger P, Klein G (1995) Laparoscopic pelvic lymph node dissection combined with real-time interactive transrectal ultrasound guided transperineal radioactive seed implantation of the prostate. J Urol 153:1555–1560
25. Klän R, Meier T, Knispel HH, Wegner HEH, Miller K (1995) Laparoscopic pelvic lymphadenectomy in prostatic cancer: analysis of seventy consecutive cases. Urol Int 55:78–83
26. Brant LA, Brant WO, Brown MH, Seid DL, Allen Jr RE (1996) A new minimally invasive open pelvic lymphadenectomy surgical technique for the staging of prostate cancer. Urology 47:416–421
27. Effert P, Boeckmann W, Wolff J, Jakse G (1996) Laparoskopische Lymphadenektomie beim Prostatakarzinom. Urologe A 35:413–417
28. Parra RO, Isorna S, Perez MG, Cummings JM, Boullier JA (1996) Radical perineal prostatectomy without pelvic lymphadenectomy: selection criteria and early results. J Urol 155:612–615
29. Cadeddu JA, Elashry OM, Snyder O, Schulam P, Moore RG, Loughlin KR, Winfield HN, Clayman RV, Kavoussi LR (1997) Effect of laparoscopic pelvic lymph node dissection on the natural history of D1 (T1-3, N1-3, M0) prostate cancer. Urology 50:391–394
30. Fahlenkamp D, Müller W, Schönberger B, Loening SA (1997) Laparoskopische Lymphadenektomie (LPLA) in der Diagnostik des lokoregionären Prostatakarzinoms. Akt Urol 28:35–42
31. Hoenig DM, Chi S, Porter C, Tackett L, Smith DS, Cohen SI, Stein BS (1997) Risk of nodal metastases at laparoscopic pelvic lymphadenectomy using PSA, Gleason score, and clinical stage in men with localized prostate cancer. J Endourol 11:263–265
32. Lemer SE, Taub HC, Fleischmann J, Chamberlin JW, Kahan N, Melman A (1994) Combined laparoscopic pelvic lymph node dissection and modified belt radical perineal prostatectomy for localized prostatic carcinoma. Urology 43:493–498

33. Paul DB, Loening SA, Narayana AS, Culp DA (1983) Morbidity from pelvic lymphadenectomy in staging carcinoma of the prostate. J Urol 129:1141–1144

34. Davis GL (1995) Sensitivity of frozen section examination of pelvic lymph nodes for metastatic prostate carcinoma. Cancer 76:661–668

35. Catalona WJ, Stein AJ (1982) Accuracy of fresh frozen section detection of lymph node metastases in prostatic carcinoma. J Urol 127:460–461

36. Rukstalis DB, Chodak GW (1992) Laparoscopic retroperitoneal lymph node dissection in a patient with stage 1 testicular carcinoma. J Urol 148:1907–1910

37. Gerber GS, Bissada NK, Hulbert JC, Kavoussi LR, Moore RG, Kantoff PW, Rukstalis DB (1994) Laparoscopic retroperitoneal lymphadenectomy: multi-institutional analysis. J Urol 152:1188–1192

38. Janetschek G, Hobsch A, Holtl L, Bartsch G (1996) Retroperitoneal lymphadenectomy for clinical stage I nonseminomatous testicular tumor: laparoscopy versus open surgery and impact of learning curve. J Urol 156:89–94

39. Rassweiler JJ, Seemann O, Henkel TO, Stock C, Frede T, Alken P (1996) Laparoscopic retroperitoneal lymph node dissection for nonseminomatous germ cell tumors: indications and limitations. J Urol 156:1108–1113

40. Bowsher WG, Clarke A, Clarke DG, Costello AJ (1992) Laparoscopic pelvic lymph node dissection. Br J Urol 70:276–279

41. Ovesen H, Iversen P, Beier-Holgersen R, Hald T, Rasmussen F, Steven K (1993) Extraperitoneal pelvioscopy in staging of bladder carcinoma and detection of pelvic lymph node metastasis. Scand J Urol Nephrol 27:211–214

42. Villers A, Vannier JL, Abecassis R, Baron JC, Anidjar M, Khoury R, Delmas V, Desmonts JM, Boccon-Gibod L (1993) Extraperitoneal endosurgical lymphadenectomy with insufflation in the staging of bladder and prostate cancer. J Endourol 7:229–235

43. Prasad BR, Parr NJ, Fowler JW (1994) Laparoscopic pelvic lymphadenectomy-early results. Br J Urol 73:271–274

44. Lang GS, Ruckle HC, Hadley HR, Lui PD, Stewart SC (1994) One hundred consecutive laparoscopic pelvic lymph node dissections: comparing complications of the first 50 cases to the second 50 cases. Urology 44:221–225

45. Puppo P, Perachino M, Ricciotti G, Carmignani G, Maffezzini M (1994) Laparoscopic pelvic lymph node dissection for prostate and bladder cancer: indication techniques and results. Arch Ital Urol Androl 66:117–123

46. Poulsen J, Krarup T (1995) Pelvic lymphadenectomy (staging) in patients with bladder cancer laparoscopic versus open approach. Scand J Urol Nephrol Suppl 172:19–21

Impact of Laparoscopy in Malignant Lymphomas

G.B. Mann · K.C. Conlon

Introduction and Background

Staging laparotomy was initially advocated from the late 1960s for patients with Hodgkin's disease (HD), and some patients with non-Hodgkin's lymphoma (NHL), to identify those patients who were potentially curable with radiotherapy and to accurately plan radiotherapy fields [1]. These procedures provided considerable information on the patterns and distribution of these diseases, altering the clinical staging in a significant group of patients [2–5]. However, the role of laparotomy has been reduced with the introduction of computerized tomographic (CT) scanning and CT-directed percutaneous biopsy, the development of combination chemotherapy, and the increased use of combined modality therapy as well as the recognition of the morbidity of laparotomy [6–8]. The degree to which the role of laparotomy has diminished because the extra information gained has been rendered redundant by new treatment protocols or, alternatively, whether protocols have been developed excluding such information because of the associated morbidity is unclear.

Since the late 1980s, minimal access surgery changed oncological surgical management significantly [9, 10]. In lymphoma, laparoscopy or peritoneoscopy has been used for many years, but it has mainly been used to direct liver biopsy to specific sites [1]. Recent development of more sophisticated instruments has allowed the surgeon to reach most parts of the abdominal cavity, including the retroperitoneum, and to biopsy areas that were previously inaccessible [11]. Dissection of suspicious tissue can provide specimens adequate for all necessary diagnostic tests, and multiple suspicious lymph nodes can be dissected [12, 13]. As a result, the role of the surgeon in assessment of abdominal lymphoma has recently been reassessed.

Several recent series suggest that minimal access surgery offers the potential to safely improve the accuracy of lymphoma diagnosis and staging, allowing treatment to be accurately tailored to the individual patient's disease [14–16]. A role for laparoscopy is emerging in diagnosis of new and recurrent lymphadenopathy, in staging patients with histologically confirmed lymphoma, and in assessment of treatment responses. A particular indication is where percutaneous biopsy has yielded inadequate information.

Role of Laparoscopy in Diagnosis

Management of patients with HD and NHL is critically dependent on an accurate pathological diagnosis. The role of surgery in providing tissue for diagnosis is clear for superficial lymphadenopathy. For intra-abdominal pathology, diagnostic options are image-guided percutaneous biopsy, open surgery, or laparoscopy. Image-guided biopsy has increased because of its relative ease and availability and because of concern about the morbidity of laparotomy and surgery-induced delay of definitive therapy.

The diagnosis of metastatic carcinoma with percutaneous fine needle aspiration (FNA) biopsy can be extremely accurate, with false positive and negative rates as low as 1% being reported [17]. Diagnosis of lymphoproliferative disorders has been more challenging than that of metastatic epithelial malignancy, however, as it can be difficult to distinguish low-grade lymphomas from reactive processes and intermediate- and high-grade lymphomas from anaplastic carcinoma, resulting in lower diagnostic accuracy [17].

Immunohistochemistry can improve the accuracy of FNA for lymphoma, with false positives almost eliminated and inconclusive or false negative rates reduced to about 10% [17, 18]. However, nodal architecture is important for distinguishing indolent from aggressive lymphomas, and this information is unavailable from FNA cytology [18]. Furthermore, cytogenetic and molecular evaluation for nonrandom genetic rearrangements can have important prognostic significance both at initial diagnosis and at relapse [19–24]; percutaneous biopsy provides inadequate tissue for such analysis.

A series of 101 laparoscopic procedures in patients from the lymphoma service at Memorial Sloan-Kettering Cancer Center [14], New York, resulted in a diagnosis of lymphoma in 62 patients with only one false negative and one technical failure (Table 1). In all cases where lymphoma was diagnosed, the biopsy specimens were adequate to allow a comprehensive diagnosis, including architecture, grade, and cell type, allowing appropriate treatment planning. A group from Lille, France reported 118 patients having retroperitoneoscopy (RPS) for retroperitoneal lymphadenopathy [15]. The overall sensitivity was 91%, but there were 9 false negatives in the 70 cases of lymphoma. Another multi-institutional series from Udine, Italy, and Los Angeles compared open and laparoscopic staging of HD [16]. The laparoscopic series were oncologically equivalent and functionally superior.

Accuracy of FNA is influenced by the clinical setting in which it is used, with better results reported for diagnosis of recurrent disease rather than for initial diagnosis [25]. Reports of FNA or core-needle biopsy in lymphoma indicate that between 72% and 86% of biopsied patients with a definite or suspicious diagnosis of lymphoma were treated on the basis of the biopsy result [25–27]. In a review of NHL, 57% (31/54) of patients without a prior history of lymphoma and 90% (35/39) of patients with a previous diagnosis of lymphoma were treated on the basis of percutaneous biopsy results alone. In 39% (12/31) of cases without a past history and in 57% (20/35) of cases with that history the pathology report was incomplete, in that it did not give an unequivocal diagnosis of lymphoma with determination of grade [25]. This suggests that in some patients therapeutic

Table 1. Indications and pathological outcomes from laparoscopy for suspected lymphoma (from [14])

Indication for laparoscopy		Number of cases		
		Total	Neoplastic diagnosis	Nonneoplastic diagnosis
Diagnosis	Abdominal mass	48	36	12
	Possible relapse	21	18	3
	Poor response/residual mass	8	6	2
	Liver biopsy	8	2	6
Staging	Abnormal CT/LAG	9	3	6
	Liver biopsy	7	4	3

decisions are being made on incomplete information, because the risks involved in obtaining further tissue are considered too great for any additional benefit.

In general, FNA is able to confirm the diagnosis of recurrent intra-abdominal lymphoma [25–27], and so it is not surprising that most patients are treated on the basis of the cytology. However, this information could be misleading if there was frequent discordance between the initial diagnosis and the repeat biopsy. The series from Memorial Sloan-Kettering suggests that this may occur in a significant minority of cases. There were 24 patients with a prior full diagnosis of lymphoma in whom the laparoscopy revealed lymphoma. In five of these patients (21%) there was a significant change in diagnosis; this was a change in lymphoma grade (3 cases), a change from HD to NHL (1 case), or a change in low-grade histology (1 case). In another case, there was a change in high-grade histology that was not clinically important.

Laparoscopic Biopsy After Previous Attempts

Laparoscopy has an obvious role when percutaneous biopsy has either been attempted or has failed to reach a diagnosis, or when the radiologist considers that the lesion is inaccessible. Of the Memorial cases, 27 patients had previously undergone a variety of procedures to obtain abdominal tissue for diagnosis. These specimens were considered nondiagnostic in ten cases, suggestive for or diagnostic of lymphoma but without adequate detail for treatment decisions in ten cases, and suspicious for other neoplasia in seven cases. After laparoscopic biopsy, 21 patients were noted to have lymphoma with sufficient detail for treatment decisions, 3 had other neoplastic conditions, and 3 did not have neoplastic conditions [14]. Similarly, 74 of the 118 patients from Lille had an FNA before retroperitoneoscopy [15].

▌ Staging

Traditionally, staging laparotomy was used to plan therapy for patients with potential intra-abdominal lymphoma. The series from Udine suggests that laparoscopic staging can provide all the information previously supplied by laparotomy [16]. Laparotomy has been largely superseded by noninvasive staging with CT scanning and/or lymphangiogram (LAG) [6-8]. For many years, LAG was the „gold standard" in the noninvasive evaluation of HD, but it too is being used less frequently, because it may not significantly add to CT staging [28-31]. Nine of the Memorial patients with an established diagnosis of extra-abdominal lymphoma underwent laparoscopy because of equivocal CT or LAG (Fig. 1) to clarify the stage and extent of treatment. Six of these patients had benign biopsies, and three showed lymphoma. Four of the five patients with equivocal or suspicious LAG proved to have benign lymph nodes.

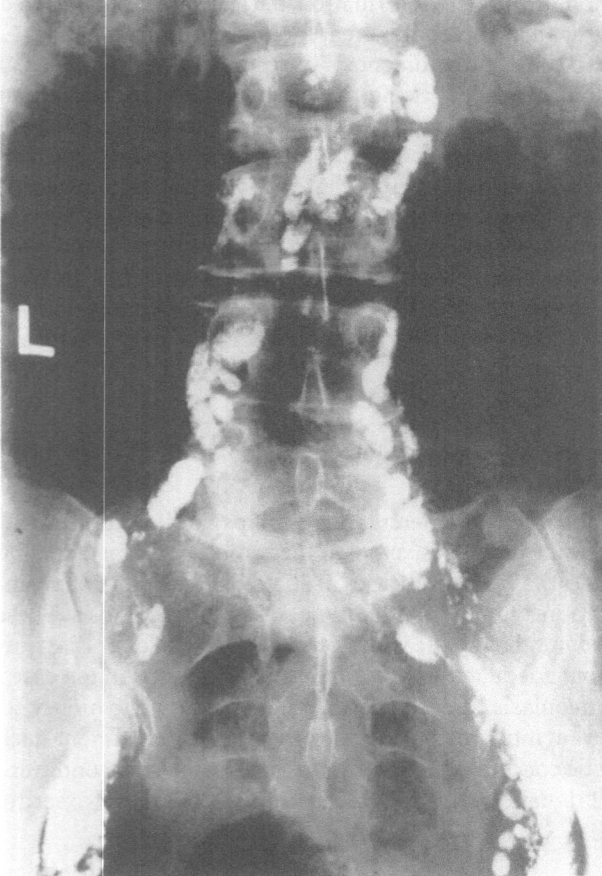

Fig. 1. Abnormal lymphangiogram demonstrating suspicious nodes along aorta

Residual Disease

The importance of residual abdominal masses in NHL after combination chemotherapy has been controversial. Up to 40% of patients with an abdominal mass at diagnosis will have a residual mass at clinical complete remission. Open biopsy revealed no evidence of residual disease in between 80% and 95% [32, 33]. These results can support either the use of restaging laparotomy to assess the true remission status [32] or a policy of observation for patients with stable masses who are otherwise in complete remission [33]. In the series from Memorial, two of the four biopsies performed to investigate a residual or persistent mass after chemotherapy showed lymphoma whereas in the other two cases the biopsies were benign. In addition, all four patients with suspected progressive disease had this confirmed on biopsy. Laparoscopic assessment of the residual mass without the morbidity of open surgery may alter management algorithms in such situations.

Impact on Treatment

The clinical impact of laparoscopy in lymphoma management was assessed in the MSKCC study (Table 2). Most of the procedures were assessed as having impact. Procedures were included as having an impact on therapy if they resulted in a pathological diagnosis or alteration or clarification in disease stage sufficient for a treatment decision. In 65 of 69 cases where the indication was to investigate a lesion for which the differential diagnosis included either a primary or recurrent lymphoma, adequate tissue was obtained to make a full diagnosis and for treatment planning. The laparoscopy was considered to have had an impact in all these cases. In all cases where the indication was to assess either a residual mass after therapy or a hepatic lesion in a lymphoma patient, the result guided treatment decisions. Where it was used to complete intra-abdominal staging in the setting of an abnormal CT or LAG, six of nine patients had benign biopsies and therefore had primary radiation therapy. The other three patients had intra-abdominal disease, and therefore needed combination therapy.

In the French series, 34 of the patients' clinical diagnosis was radically changed by the results of RPS, including 30 patients suspected to have lymphoma, who turned out to have a variety of benign and malignant conditions.

Assessment of impact from retrospective reviews of medical records can at best give an approximate guide, but from these reports it is clear that minimal access surgery has a definite role to play.

Table 2. Clinical impact of the laparoscopic procedures (from [14])

Indication	Description of clinical result		n	Impact (%)
Diagnosis	Abdominal mass	Treated on basis of neoplastic biopsy	34	45/48
		Neoplastic biopsy, no effect on treatment	2[a]	(94)
		Benign biopsy: true negative	11	
		False negative	0	
		No diagnosis from biopsy	1[a]	
	Possible relapse	Treated on basis of neoplastic biopsy	18	20/21
		Benign biopsy: true negative	2	(95)
		False negative	1[a]	
	Poor response or residual mass	Further treatment after positive biopsy	6	6/6
		No further treatment after negative biopsy	2	(100)
	Liver biopsy	Treatment altered after positive biopsy	2	8/8
		Exclusion of lymphomatous involvement	6	(100)
Staging	Abnormal CT/LAG	More extensive treatment after positive biopsy	3	9/9
		Confirmation of limited-stage disease	6	(100)
	Liver biopsy	Up- or down-staging altering treatment plan	4	4/7
		Positive or negative biopsy with no clinical impact	3	(57)

[a]Indicates categories where procedure was deemed to have had no impact.

Technical Aspects

Various approaches have been used for endoscopic biopsy in lymphoma. Peritoneoscopy to guide liver biopsy has been replaced by multiport laparoscopy. This has allowed access to all parts of the peritoneal cavity, as well as many retroperitoneal structures (Fig. 2). RPS is an alternative approach to that area.

The report from Memorial Sloan-Kettering emphasized the importance of high-quality preoperative imaging from accurate surgical planning and also the benefit of intraoperative frozen section analysis to maximize the diagnostic yield. In the French series, on the other hand, no frozen section analysis was used, and a much lower sensitivity was reported, with a 12% false negative rate. In addition, nodes are removed intact as far as possible to maximize the diagnostic yield (Figs. 3, 4). Use of titanium clips for hemostasis allowed postoperative confirmation that the correct tissue had been biopsied.

In the Memorial series, only 3 of the 101 procedures were completed by open surgery after laparoscopy yielded inadequate samples. Morbidity for the laparo-

Fig. 2. Retroperitoneum exposed (same patient as in Fig. 1)

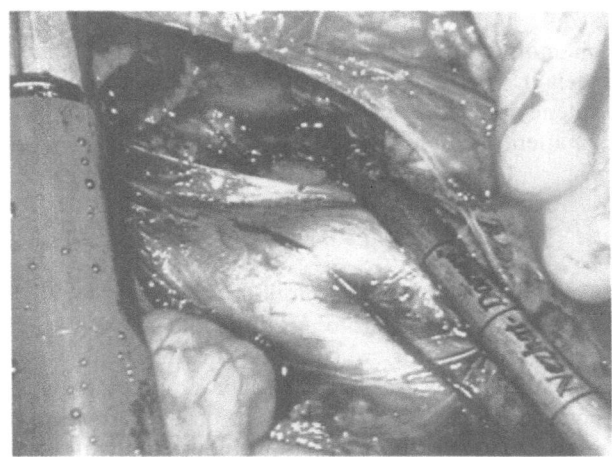

Fig. 3. Periportal adenopathy in a patient after chemotherapy for HD

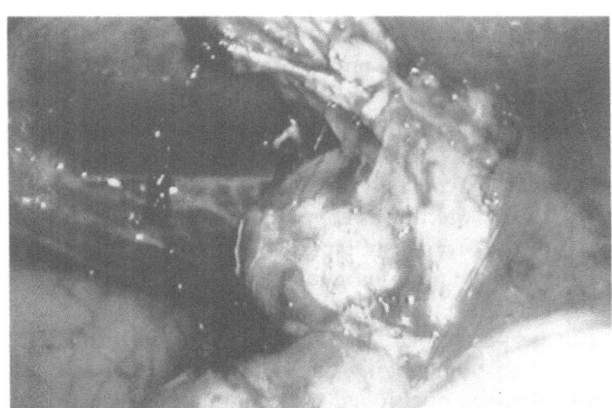

Fig. 4. Complete excision of lymph node

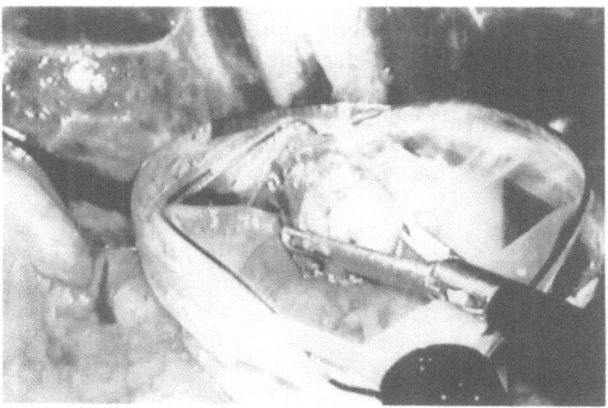

scopic procedure was minimal, and many patients commenced definitive chemotherapy within days of the diagnostic procedure [14]. Similar results were seen in the other series, with the main complication being bleeding during splenectomy in 2 of 15 cases from Udine [16] and bleeding from lumbar veins in 2 patients from Lille [15].

Conclusion and Future Directions

The advent of combined modality treatment for malignant lymphomas has resulted in staging laparotomy falling into disuse [34]. Current diagnostic and therapeutic algorithms are based on the historical evidence of high morbidity and mortality that were seen with laparotomy and splenectomy. Laparoscopic surgery has been shown to be able to provide adequate tissue for complete analysis in most cases with minimal morbidity and without the problems involved with administration of chemotherapy during recovery from a laparotomy. Integration of laparoscopic staging may allow more precisely tailored therapy without the costs and risks of laparotomy. Until the promise of laparoscopy to provide precise data with low morbidity and minimal interruption of treatment schedules is confirmed, its role will remain uncertain. Current reports suggest that it should be considered when percutaneous biopsy is not technically possible, when chromosomal or genetic analysis is needed for treatment decisions, or when the results of CT-guided FNA are incomplete. The early use of laparoscopy in cases of possible residual or recurrent disease after chemotherapy, or when the disease does not respond to therapy as expected, can quickly clarify the situation.

For the promise of laparoscopy in lymphoma to be realized, therapeutic algorithms for lymphoma management will have to be reassessed. This will require the current reports that tissue biopsies from specific intra-abdominal locations can be performed with minimal morbidity to be confirmed in many centers. Oncologists managing lymphoma who have access to high-quality laparoscopy will then be positioned to recommend precisely tailored therapy for their patients confident that the diagnosis is complete and accurate. A recent report of the superiority of combined chemoradiation over chemotherapy alone for localized high- and intermediate-grade NHL [35] was accompanied by a commentary describing three general approaches: chemotherapy alone, combined treatment, or investigation to determine which is best [36]. Laparoscopy seems to offer safe, accurate, and comprehensive diagnostic capabilities and so should be considered in this schema.

References

1. Glatstein E, Guernsey JM, Rosenberg SA, et al (1969) The value of laparotomy and splenectomy in the staging of Hodgkin's disease. Cancer 24:709–718
2. Veronesi U, Musumeci R, Pizzetti F, Gennari L, Bonnadonna G (1974) The value of staging laparotomy in non-Hodgkins lymphoma. Cancer 33:446–459
3. Chabner BA, Johnson RE, Young RL, Cannellos GP, Hubbard SP, Johnson SK, DeVita VT (1976) Sequential nonsurgical and surgical staging of non-Hodgkin's lymphoma. Ann Int Med 85:149–154
4. Goffinet DR, Warnke R, Dunnick NR, Castellino R, Platstein E, Nelson TS, Dorfman RF, Rosenberg SA, Kaplan HS (1977) Clinical and surgical (laparotomy) evaluation of patients with non-Hodgkin's lymphoma. Cancer Treatment Reports 61:981–992
5. Heifetz L, Fuller L, Rodgers R, et al (1980) Laparotomy findings in lymphangiogram staged I and II Non-Hodgkin's Lymphomas. Cancer 45:2778
6. Meeker WR, Richardson JD, West WO, et al (1972) Critical evaluation of laparotomy and splenectomy in Hodgkin's disease. Arch Surg 105:222–229
7. Desser RK, Ultmann JE (1972) Risk of severe infection in patients with Hodgkin's disease or lymphoma after diagnostic laparotomy and splenectomy (editorial). Ann Intern Med 77:143–146
8. Lacher MJ (1983) Routine staging laparotomy for patients with Hodgkin's disease is no longer necessary. Cancer Invest 1:93–99
9. Conlon KC, Docherty E, Klimstra DS, et al (1996) The value of minimal access surgery in the staging of patients with potentially resectable peripancreatic malignancy. Ann Surg 223:134–140
10. Conlon KC, Karpeh MS Jr. (1996) Laparoscopy and laparoscopic ultrasound in the staging of gastric cancer. Semin Oncol 23:347–351
11. Salky BA, Bauer JJ, Gelernt IM, et al (1988) The use of laparoscopy in retroperitoneal pathology. Gastrointest Endosc 34:227–230
12. Rassweiler JJ, Seemann O, Henkel TO, et al (1996) Laparoscopic retroperitoneal lymph node dissection for nonseminomatous germ cell tumors: indications and limitations. J Urology 156:1108–1113
13. Gerber GS, Rukstalis DB (1996) Laparoscopic approach to retroperitoneal lymph node dissection. Semin Surg Oncol 12:121–125
14. Mann GB, Conlon KC, LaQuaglia M, Dougherty E, Moskowitz C, Zelenetz A (1998) Emerging role for laparoscopy in the diagnosis of lymphoma. J Clin Oncol 16:1909–1915
15. Porte H, Copin MC, Eraldi L, Roumilhac D, Jaillard-Thery S, Puech P, Bauters F, Gosselin B, Wurtz A (1997) Retinoscopy for the diagnosis of infiltrating retroperitoneal lymphadenopathy and masses. Br J Surg 84:1433–1436
16. Baccarani U, Carroll BJ, Hiatt JR, Donini A, Terrosu G, Decker R, Chandra M, Basadola F, Phillips EH (1998) Comparison of laparoscopic and open staging in Hodgkin's disease. Arch Surg 133:517–522
17. Steel BL, Schwartz MR, Ramzy I (1994) Fine needle aspiration biopsy in the diagnosis of lymphadenopathy in 1,103 patients. Acta Cytol 38:76–81
18. Sneige N, Dekmezian RH, Katz RL, et al (1990) Morphologic and immunocytochemical evaluation of 220 fine needle aspirates of malignant lymphoma and lymphoid hyperplasia. Acta Cytol 34:311–322
19. Yunis JJ, Mayer MG, Arnesen MA, et al (1989) *bcl*-2 and other genomic alterations in the prognosis of large-cell lymphoma. N Engl J Med 320:1047–1054
20. Hardy R, Horning SJ (1991) Molecular biologic studies in the clinical evaluation of non-Hodgkin's lymphoma. Hematol Oncol Clin North Am 5:891–900

21. Offit K, Lo Coco F, Louie DC, et al (1994) Rearrangement of the *bcl-6* gene as a prognostic marker in diffuse large-cell lymphoma. New Engl J Med 331:74–80

22. Tilly H, Rossi A, Stamatoullas A, et al (1994) Prognostic value of chromosomal abnormalities in follicular lymphoma. Blood 84:1043–1049

23. Bastard C, Deweindt C, Kerckaert JP, et al (1994) LAZ3 rearrangements in non-Hodgkin's lymphoma: correlation with histology, immunophenotype, karyotype and clinical outcome in 217 patients. Blood 83:2423–2427

24. Offit K, Louie DC, Parsa NZ, et al (1995) BCL6 gene rearrangement and other cytogenetic abnormalities in diffuse large cell lymphoma. Leukemia and Lymphoma 20:85–89

25. Silverman SG, Lee BY, Mueller PR, et al (1994) Impact of positive findings at image-guided biopsy of lymphoma on patient care: evaluation of clinical history, needle size, and pathological findings on biopsy performance. Radiology 190:759–764

26. Pappa VI, Hussain HK, Reznek RH, et al (1996) Role of image-guided core-needle biopsy in the management of patients with lymphoma. J Clin Oncol 14:2427–2430

27. Ben-Yehuda D, Polliack A, Okan E, et al (1996) Image-guided core-needle biopsy in malignant lymphoma: experience with 100 patients that suggests the technique is reliable. J Clin Oncol 14:2431–2434

28. Castellino RA, Hoppe RT, Blank N, et al (1984) Computed tomography, lymphography, and staging laparotomy: correlations in initial staging of Hodgkin disease. AJR 143:37–41

29. Marglin S, Castellino R (1981) Lymphographic accuracy in 632 consecutive, previously untreated cases of Hodgkin disease and non-Hodgkin lymphoma. Radiology 140:351–353

30. Musemeci R, Tesoso-Tess JD (1994) New imaging techniques in staging lymphomas. Curr Opin Oncol 6:464–469

31. North LB, Wallace S, Lindell MM, et al (1993) Lymphography for staging lymphomas: Is it still a useful procedure? AJR 161:867–869

32. Surbane A, Longo DL, DeVita VT, et al (1988) Residual abdominal masses in aggressive non-Hodgkin's lymphoma after combination chemotherapy: significance and management. J Clin Oncol 6:1832–1837

33. Fuks JZ, Aisner J, Wiernik PH (1982) Restaging laparotomy in the management of the non-Hodgkin's lymphomas. Med Pediatr Oncol 10:429–438

34. Bonnadonna G (1994) Modern treatment of malignant lymphomas: A multidisciplinary approach? Ann Oncol 5:S5–S16

35. Miller TP, Dahlberg JR, Cassady JR, et al (1998) Chemotherapy alone compared with chemotherapy plus radiotherapy for localized intermediate- and high-grade non-Hodgkin's lymphoma. N Engl J Med 339:21–26

36. Cosset JM (1998) Chemoradiotherapy for localized non-Hodgkin's lymphoma. N Engl J Med 339:44–45

Subject-Index